Praise for *Why Smart People Make Bad Food Choices*

"*Why Smart People Make Bad Food Choices* exposes the tragic ways our minds and environment conspire to undermine our nutritional health. Jack Bobo takes the reader on a fascinating journey into the latest research in psychology and behavior to offer a realistic alternative to fad diets and pop science to address obesity in America. If you've ever wondered why it's so hard to make good food choices and what could be done to make it easier, do yourself a favor and read this book."

—**Michiel Bakker**, vice president of workforce spaces at Google

"The tide of obesity in America is rising with staggering health consequences. Meeting the daily requirement for calories and nutrients is so seemingly simple, yet so fraught with complexity. Jack Bobo's investigation of the science and psychology behind our food choices shines a light on why we behave the way we do and proposes a path to a healthier future."

—**Kathryn Boor**, PhD, dean and vice provost of graduate education at Cornell University

"Almost all of us eat almost every day. That may make us feel like experts—but familiarity is not expertise. Our food and diet relate to our family, religion, childhood memories, culture, economy, environmental beliefs, social interactions, and health. With so many connections, it is no wonder there is so much public attention to food and diet, so many opinions offered, so much public conflict and dispute about diet and food. There is no shortage of information (or perhaps more aptly, myth, presumption, and misinformation)— there is a glut. How can the intelligent, interested person who wants to base their beliefs or ⋯⋯ ⋯ of this

T0150760

morass? Jack Bobo is one of an emerging choir of guiding voices of rationality. Bobo is a modern polymath—a legal scholar, nutritionist, environmentalist, and thought leader. He conveys an enormous breadth of fascinating research findings in this new book. Yet, he is at least as much provocateur as rapporteur. He challenges common misconceptions and asks the reader to think anew, to think broadly, and, perhaps most of all, to think big. His billion-calorie project exemplifies this much-needed big-thinking as we consider 'One-Health' accepting responsibility not only for our own health, but also for that of our planet."

—**David B. Allison**, PhD, distinguished professor, obesity and nutrition researcher, and academic dean

"Inadequate food choices leading to health disorders like obesity are not just a problem of rich countries. It constitutes the double burden of nutrition worldwide: the coexistence of under-nutrition and over-nutrition. Based on a detailed analysis of the psychological and environmental mechanisms in the US, Jack Bobo shows the enormous risks for every country. It is a call for action, everywhere."

—**Louise O. Fresco**, president of the Wageningen University and Research executive board

"Obesity is a crisis that must be addressed urgently. Rich developed nations are killing themselves with too much food whilst, elsewhere in the world, people are dying for want of it. The current Covid pandemic has shone a light on the high morbidity amongst the obese and so everything must be done to empower citizens to reclaim the healthy bodies they need. Insights into why we make bad food choices and how that could change is to be welcomed."

—**Professor Dame Anne Glover**, FRS FRSE, president of the Royal Society of Edinburgh, special advisor at the University of Strathclyde, and former chief scientific adviser to the European Commission

"In *Why Smart People Make Bad Food Choices*, Jack Bobo exposes the not-so-obvious but real drivers of our complicated relationship to the foods we choose and why it's proven so hard to change our poor eating habits. Only then does it become apparent why our current approaches haven't worked and how genuine and achievable solutions can be found. This book is an essential read for those of us trying to understand the mysteries behind the food choices and eating habits of today's consumer."

—**Stephen M Ostroff**, MD, former deputy commissioner for Foods and Veterinary Medicine, FDA

WHY
Smart
People

MAKE

Bad
Food
Choices

The Invisible Influences
that Guide Our Thinking

WHY
Smart
People

MAKE

Bad
Food
Choices

The Invisible Influences
that Guide Our Thinking

Jack A Bobo

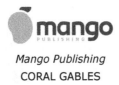

Mango Publishing
CORAL GABLES

Cover & Layout Design: Carmen Fortunato
Cover Photo: Adobe Stock
Illustrations: ©2021 David West Reynolds/Phaeton Group
Author Photograph: by TBD
Editorial services by Phaeton Group Science Media www.phaetongroup.com

For permission requests, please contact the publisher at:
Mango Publishing Group
2850 S Douglas Road, 2nd Floor
Coral Gables, FL 33134 USA
info@mango.bz

For special orders, quantity sales, course adoptions and corporate sales, please email the publisher at sales@mango.bz. For trade and wholesale sales, please contact Ingram Publisher Services at customer.service@ingramcontent.com or +1.800.509.4887.

Why Smart People Make Bad Food Choices: The Invisible Influences that Guide Our Thinking

Library of Congress Cataloging-in-Publication number: 2021934499
ISBN: (print) 978-1-64250-592-4, (ebook) 978-1-64250-593-1
BISAC category code HEA006000, HEALTH & FITNESS / Diet & Nutrition / Diets

Printed in the United States of America

DISCLAIMER:
Although the author and publisher have made every effort to ensure that the information in this book was correct at press time, the author and publisher do not assume and hereby disclaim any liability to any party for any loss, damage, or disruption caused by errors or omissions, whether such errors or omissions result from negligence, accident, or any other cause. This book is not intended as a substitute for the medical advice of physicians, registered dietitians, nutritionists, or other health care professionals. Readers should consult with qualified health care professionals in matters relating to their health.

For my wife Qiao,
my harshest critic and my biggest fan

Contents

Foreword

By Esther Dyson

Welcome to *Why Smart People Make Bad Food Choices*!
If you're smart, this book is for you!

Just kidding... But seriously, my hope is not for everyone to read this book. My hope is for it to be unnecessary, because our society will make it easy for everyone to make smart food choices and smart health choices in general. I write as the executive founder of Wellville. net, a ten-year nonprofit project devoted to helping five small US communities turn themselves into healthier and more equitable places to grow up and live.

The book is full of useful ideas and context, but it's not directed primarily at individuals; rather, it's for people like those we work with directly at Wellville: people who have influence over the environment that governs so much of our behavior. It's mostly useless to give individuals advice if they encounter too many obstacles to following it. Yes, people should not go on diets forced-march style. They should eat and exercise every day as a matter of course, because it is convenient and feels good. Personally, I would hate to have to decide to go swimming every day. Too much cognitive overload. Instead, if I'm traveling and cannot go to my Y a convenient ten-minute walk nearby, I just need to figure out how. In short: it's not that I decide to swim. I'm a daily swimmer; it's part of my identity.

So is my reluctance to put junk into my body; I have too many important things to do to be consumed by lassitude or a sugar surge. (And FWIW, I'm more concerned with sugar than with fat, the one point where Jack and I might disagree.)

But I'm really lucky: I can afford healthy food, I live near a top-notch YMCA, and I don't have kids to take care of or a job with inconvenient hours that doesn't pay me enough to buy the food I'd prefer. Those are all the environmental affordances that make it possible for me to be so annoyingly healthy…and they are what this book is about. Most people are not so lucky—and that's reflected in the alarming rate of obesity, diabetes, and related ills in this country (and increasingly in the world).

It's not a book about prescriptions or recipes as much as it is about the ingredients that can make it possible for a community—not just individuals—to stay healthy and build resilience. That resilience is an asset that can help people to deal with the inevitable challenges of life, whether that's a distressing death in the family, the rigors of a new job or a new baby, a COVID-19 lockdown, or COVID-19 itself.

That is why I founded Wellville. Wellville's five communities signed up to become healthier; it's not as if I, a nice white lady, showed up to tell them what to do. They are real places, not a new construction.

That means that, like most people, these communities have a lot of "pre-existing conditions": de facto segregation, schools of varying quality, poverty, politics, shortages of time and agency… There's so much to fix. The challenge is not creating new communities from scratch; it's helping real places heal and prosper.

Many people in these communities don't have it easy, but many have learned to thrive despite the obstacles. Our role is to help those who thrive reach out to help others to thrive as well, reshaping both a healthier culture and healthier institutions.

This book can be a tremendous help for those looking to reshape their food systems for the better. But many of its lessons—around thought patterns, around long-term thinking, around collaboration—hold true for other issues as well.

Just to be concrete, here are some of the ways we at Wellville hope to see our communities put these ideas to work. Much of Jack's advice in this book is directly relevant.

The *tactic* is to support the community in demanding an environment and services that will make it easy to eat right, exercise, and live free of constant anxiety.

The *strategy* is to round up a variety of vendors to help meet that demand in a variety of ways, and also to find some long-term-thinking funders (including insurers and employers as well as grant-makers) to fund/subsidize some of the interventions as necessary. We're also hoping that they will see long-term business returns—and that insurers will fund interventions based on outcomes.

In addition, we hope to see the healthcare systems cooperating with a variety of community organizations to make healthcare less necessary! That sounds alarming, but it will give the healthcare providers more capacity to deal with severe illnesses, as well as the ability to offer checkups and preventive care, when they operate in a community where preventable illness is rare.

Indeed, the *goal* is to help the community become a healthier place to grow up and live in. We are hoping for a lot of *second-hand impact*; that is, for every person who participates actively in some kind of intervention, some additional number will be affected without signing up for a "program." That will happen both among community members/employees as individuals, and within individuals as consumers/users of food and public facilities (among other things).

So, dear reader, over to you! You can't generally succeed by telling people what to do, but you can certainly make it easier for them to follow good advice!

Introduction

Why is it that at a time when people have never known more about health and nutrition, they have never been more obese? We ignore recommendations to eat less and exercise more and instead collectively spend billions of dollars on fad diets that, deep down, we know will not deliver results. In other words, why do smart people make bad food choices?

From superfoods to clean eating, we are seduced by marketing pitches that inevitably fail to deliver lasting results. Even worse, some diet fads can produce real harm, as was the case with one New York City "wellness" blogger. In 2014, Jordan Younger was living the influencer dream with her 70,000 Instagram followers. She described herself as a "gluten-free, sugar-free, oil-free, grain-free, legume-free, plant-based, raw vegan." She believed she was eating the healthiest of all possible diets. She shared her wisdom through social media and books, and despite Younger not having any qualifications as a nutritionist, her message was popular: 40,000 people bought copies of her twenty-five-dollar, five-day "cleanse" program.

Younger was meticulously following the "clean" diet she promoted up until the day she noticed her hair falling out. Unfortunately for Younger, her dedication to "clean" eating had veered into an obsession, and the diet she was hawking was actually making her extremely ill. Younger eventually realized her error, and in 2015, she wrote a memoir, *Breaking Vegan*, that chronicled her self-destructive fixation with "clean eating" and her obsessive focus on "healthy," "unprocessed" foods. She had become a cautionary tale for fad diets. (But don't worry about her. Her health bounced back, and her following returned after a little rebranding. With a new set of diet recommendations, she offers podcasts and recipes as "The Balanced Blonde," and she now has nearly 230,000 Instagram followers.)

Younger's story may be extreme, but with 42 percent of Americans obese and the number rising, the desire to find a healthier path is something we can all relate to. Bookstore shelves are lined with self-help books promoting "simple tricks" to a healthy lifestyle, and grocery store aisles are stocked with health foods—as well as foods with health claims, which may not actually be all that healthy, as we will see.

With so many tools available, it must all come down to willpower, right? It's hard not to conclude that the problem is us. But that would be wrong. The truth is that diets don't work for most people. Sure, many diets work for some people for a short period of time, but there just isn't much evidence that any particular diet works for most people over a period of months or years. Furthermore, the research is pretty clear that a lack of self-control is not what's making us fat. I suggest you ignore the hype about harnessing your willpower and consider some new ideas that might actually have an impact.

I grew up in a small town in Indiana. My family didn't own a farm, but we did have a large garden. We grew corn, tomatoes, peppers, green beans, onions, cantaloupes, strawberries, and probably many other things that I've forgotten. My mother canned vegetables for the winter and made jellies and jams as well. We didn't always have a lot of money when I was growing up, but always had enough to eat. Despite having plenty of food, nobody in my family gave much thought to how we were eating. My mother constantly reminded me and my brothers to eat more and we certainly weren't allowed to leave food on our plates. Even with the nagging to eat up, my brothers and I never had to worry about our weight. Neither did any of my neighbors or friends, as far as I can recall. It wasn't knowledge of healthy eating habits or nutrition that kept us thin. In fact, we never gave such things a second thought.

Reducing obesity in America is not about diets or information. It's not about reading labels or counting calories. Instead, it is about changing our food culture, which is the sum of all of our habits combined with our environment. Food culture in America has changed drastically since the 1970s, when I was growing up. And it isn't one thing, it's everything.

Diets are built on the premise that we can lose ten, twenty, or thirty pounds in months if we just stick to the plan, but that's not how we gained the weight. We gained one, two, or three pounds a year for thirty years. In order to get back to a place where knowing what and how much to eat is an afterthought rather than an act of soldierly willpower, we need to change our food habits, and to do that we need to change our food environment. If we do, we will find that we lose one, two, or three pounds a year for the next thirty years, and we'll get back to a healthier, happier way of being. It will be slow and barely noticeable along the way, but unlike most diet weight losses, this will be lasting, and it will also occur without strenuous willpower effort. If we put our effort into changing the system, then the system around us can accomplish the desired change in our bodies.

So, how do we get to a place where our habits and our food environment do the work of making us healthier?

In Part I, I will share research that proves the rather surprising fact that our brains really can't be trusted. I will examine how the cognitive biases and mental shortcuts that are hardwired into our minds often lead us to make bad food choices. If you've ever gone to the grocery store and come home with unhealthy snacks that you didn't intend to buy, then you're familiar with the impact of "decision fatigue," which is just one of many biases at work undermining our health. By recognizing these tendencies and understanding the situations in which they arise, we can take steps to limit their influence.

In Part II, I will look at the many ways our food environment exerts an invisible influence guiding our choices, often in unhealthy directions. It turns out that many of the things in our environment that we think are important, like food labels, are not as important as we think, while things like the order in which people around the table order food can be much more influential on our food choices than we ever imagined. As in Part I, understanding how our environment influences our food choices better positions us to make decisions that support our long-term goals and not simply our short-term desires.

In Part III, I consider some ways we can begin to reshape our food environment so that it no longer works against us. Drawing on lessons from behavioral science, we can redesign our food environment to deliver healthy choices. From the practical experience of companies like Google that are redesigning their workspaces to improve the food choices of their employees to the Blue Zone Projects of *National Geographic* adventurer Dan Buettner and Wellville founder Esther Dyson who are working with cities to build healthy communities, there are many exciting examples of behavioral science driving healthier food choices. This section of the book is a call to action for all of us who want to reshape our relationship with food and return to a time when food was about enjoyment and not about nutrients; when ingredients were the building blocks of a meal, not something to be scared of. By the time you finish this book, I hope you will be ready to be part of that change.

I didn't set out to write a book about how to address obesity in America. I am not a registered dietitian or a medical doctor, but this is not really a diet book at all. Instead, this is a book about how our brains lead us to make bad food choices and how our environment contributes to the problem. But it is also a book about how to bring people together to change our environment to improve our decisions. These are things I know something about.

In 2002, I went to work for the US Department of State, where I served under four Secretaries of State—Colin Powell, Condoleezza Rice, Hillary Clinton, and John Kerry. I spent the next thirteen years traveling to more than fifty countries discussing global food policy. In each country I traveled to, I had the opportunity to visit research institutes to learn about agriculture and food—Rothamsted in the United Kingdom, the Chinese Agricultural University in China, the International Rice Research Institute in the Philippines, the Commonwealth Scientific and Industrial Research Organisation in Australia, the International Institute of Tropical Agriculture in Nigeria, and many more everywhere in between.

I also learned a lot at the State Department about how people think and how to successfully build consensus to drive change. I have spent the last decade reading and writing about behavioral science and what lessons it has for improving decisions. In the works of Daniel Kahneman, Richard Thaler, Cass Sunstein, Paul Slovic, Dan Ariely, and many others, I realized that tools already existed to make the changes necessary to improve our food choices. Some of the ideas are being deployed by companies right now, and there are even efforts by a few cities, but we have not yet achieved anything near the scale we need. This book is meant to help change that. Thank you for joining me on this journey.

Part I

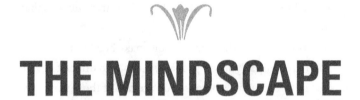

THE MINDSCAPE

Smart People Change Their Minds

I like to cook. In fact, I do a lot of the cooking in my house. I enjoy going online to find new recipes. I also like to experiment with new flavors, sometimes adding an Indian spice twist to a traditional American or Italian dish. I think I am pretty good, and my wife and children seem to agree, at least most of the time. While I do not expect to be competing on Iron Chef anytime soon, I feel confident that I am an above-average cook.

But am I really as good as I think I am? Research suggests that I might not be.

This book is about why smart people make bad food choices. Since you're reading it, you are probably curious to understand why that is the case. Perhaps it's because you are one of those smart people who sometimes makes bad food choices. Or it may be that you see smart people making bad choices all the time, even when they are warned not to.

It is pretty easy to see when the choices others make are bad for them. On the other hand, it is not nearly so obvious when we are making bad choices ourselves. One reason for this is that our brains try to protect us from disappointing news, like how we are not as great or amazing as we think we are. We are often far more confident in our own abilities than we have any right to be. Even my assessment of my cooking skills is probably too generous.

Everyone Is Above Average

Ask yourself this question: Are you an above-average driver? If you are like most people, you answered in the affirmative.

You may be familiar with the famous study that asked people to compare their driving ability to others, requiring them to rate themselves as above average, average, or below average. I don't think anyone was surprised to learn that more than 80 percent of respondents said they were above-average drivers.[1] (For what it's worth, I think of myself as an above-average driver, too.) While that outcome may be mathematically impossible, it is also pretty consistent with what we know of human behavior. We are all above average, just like the children in Garrison Keillor's fictional hometown of Lake Wobegon.

If you think it's hard to find someone who thinks they are an average driver, imagine how hard it would be to find someone who believes they are a *below*-average driver. I'm not sure such a person exists. Such self-awareness would be crushing to the soul for most of us.

Findings like these are easy to laugh at, mostly because it is hard for most of us to imagine that we might be one of those misguided individuals who are wrong about their driving skills. But remember, one in three drivers who think they are above average are wrong. Their brains just don't want to admit it.

Our hubris is not limited to our automotive skills. Most people think they are above average at most things. Studies show that people rate themselves as above average in creativity, intelligence, dependability, athleticism, honesty, friendliness, and so on. Provide people with a survey about almost any positive trait, and the vast majority will rate themselves above average. Social psychologists call it the better-than-average effect.[2]

Intellectual Humility

What does this have to do with our bad food choices, you might be wondering? As it turns out, quite a lot.

The more confident we are in the decisions we make, the less likely we are to stop and question those decisions. Even if we do take the occasional break to contemplate the possibility that we are suffering from confirmation bias, we assume that we are less likely than others to be biased.

So what are we to do?

Amazon founder Jeff Bezos sits atop one of the most successful companies of our time as well as a personal fortune of some $150 billion. I think we can all agree that by most definitions, the guy is pretty smart. But you don't run one of the largest companies in the world by yourself, no matter how smart you are. You have to surround yourself with other smart people who can help make your vision a reality.

Bezos doesn't just look for intelligent people or people who are right most of the time. For him, that is only half of the equation. He also looks for people who can admit they are wrong and who change their opinions when the situation demands. He finds that the smartest people are constantly revising their understanding and reconsidering problems they thought they had already solved. Unlike many of us who are fixed in our views, the smartest people, according to Bezos, are open to new points of view, new information, new ideas, contradictions, and challenges to their own way of thinking.[3]

That willingness to consider new information goes hand in hand with a willingness to admit that your old way of thinking was flawed. In other words—and this is the interesting part—to be super smart, you have to change your mind a lot. Bezos apparently agrees with essayist Ralph Waldo Emerson, who famously declared, "Consistency is the hobgoblin of little minds." Consistency is overrated. Bezos believes it is perfectly healthy to have a new idea tomorrow that contradicts the idea you hold today.

The Strength of Humility

Modern science agrees with both Bezos and Emerson. Psychologists refer to this flexibility of mind as "intellectual humility." Studies of decision-making show that people who are more willing to entertain the idea that they might be wrong make markedly better choices. Rather than thinking of being wrong as a sign of stupidity or ignorance, we should see it as a sign of curiosity, openness to new information and, ultimately, intelligence.[4]

In an increasingly interconnected and complicated world, the willingness to revise our views is more critical than ever. In the food sphere, we are inundated with information from every direction promising cures for all manner of ills, from superfoods that protect us from disease to diets that help us live long and happy lives. The latest scientific discoveries are amplified by the news media and then twisted and distorted until they bear little resemblance to the actual findings of the scientists who conducted the research. In this way, nutrition studies showing vague associations between some food, ingredient, or supplement and heart health in mice are promoted on the news and on social media as critical findings for public health or even miracle cures.

Good science travels quickly, but inflated or dubious information travels at the speed of light. Technology makes it easier to amplify and spread questionable information incredibly quickly. To guard against false and misleading information, we need to be both curious *and* intellectually humble.

Open Minds

I imagine many readers nodding along with the advice that we should be intellectually humble and that we should change our minds when we learn new facts. If I posed the question, "Do you consider yourself open-minded," what would you say? I imagine that nearly 100 percent of readers would agree that they are open-minded. That's the kind of person who reads a book like this, after all.

Now ask yourself: When was the last time you changed your mind? Was it last week, last month, or maybe last year? Could it be that you can't actually remember the last time you changed your mind about something important?

All of this begs the question, "Is it possible to be open-minded if you never change your mind?"

When we were children, we were exposed to new ideas and experiences all the time, and we frequently changed our minds as a result. We were encouraged to do so. In high school and college, we were taught to challenge our assumptions and to ask questions of ourselves and others. Instead of being given the answers, we learned how to seek out knowledge. Changing our minds was a sign of growth and development.

But eventually, we grow up and find careers. Our circle of friends becomes fixed. Perhaps we get married, have children, and settle down. Whether it happens in our twenties, thirties, or forties, at some point the rate at which we change our minds begins to slow and, for some, to practically stop. Rather than spend time searching for knowledge that challenges our beliefs, we look for facts that support or defend them.

Confirmation bias allows us to convince ourselves that we have carefully considered or fully vetted new ideas before we reject them. As Bishop Oldham wrote in 1906, "A great many people think they are thinking when they are merely rearranging their prejudices."[5]

As we get older, it becomes less comfortable to change our minds because we have become so invested in our old beliefs. We have surrounded ourselves with people who believe the same things that we believe. Our jobs may even depend on, or be a reflection of, our beliefs. This means there would be a cost associated with changing our minds. Better to hang onto a silly belief than to give up on an important friendship. Too often, we choose habit and comfort over growth and knowledge.

Strong Opinions, Weakly Held

There are a lot of strongly held beliefs in the food world. It only takes a few minutes on social media to find people with views on pretty much everything. Some people swear by the Keto Diet, others are followers of Atkins. Clean eating is still the rage among many, while believers in cleanses and intermittent fasting are only too eager to share the latest research supporting their dietary choices. Then there are the vegans, vegetarians, reducetarians, and pescatarians, who have their own perspectives on healthy, ethical eating. Will it be long before the Rotarians come out with their own cookbook and diet plan as well?

Following a diet or way of eating that works for you is not the problem. There are many ways of eating a healthy and nutritious diet, though we need to keep in mind that for a diet to work it must work not only for days, weeks, and months, but for a lifetime. For many, diets are like fashions—they change with the seasons.

So how do we open ourselves to new information without getting swept up in the latest fad?

Rather than throw up our hands and give up on finding real solutions, the answer may be to have "strong opinions, which are weakly held." This is the advice of futurist Bob Johansen from the Institute for the Future. Strongly held opinions give us the confidence to be decisive and make important decisions. Weakly held opinions are equally important because that means you are not too attached to what you believe. Being too attached to ideas undermines our ability to see and hear evidence that conflicts with our opinions.[6]

While Jeff Bezos may think of flexibility of the mind as a trait of the smartest people, it reminds me of the difference between smart people and wise people. Smart people are those who know a lot, but nonetheless they sometimes make bad choices, because *all* people sometimes make bad choices. Wise people are those who *learn* from their mistakes and make better choices going forward. My point is that you don't have to be a genius to be wise.

In the struggle to make better choices, our brains are sometimes working against us. Our biases often lead us in the wrong direction, particularly when it comes to food. Fortunately, we can do something about that. This book lays out many of the ways our brains trick and mislead us. Awareness of these biases and cognitive errors will greatly reduce the mischief that they cause in your life.

In order for us to make good decisions about the food we eat, we need to be willing to change our minds—about food, but also about other things in our lives as well. By entertaining the possibility that we might be wrong and embracing genuine intellectual humility, we can move past the illusions of the "better-than-average" effect and make choices that are truly better.

Chapter 1

Why We Fear the Food We Eat

Preservatives, artificial food colorings, gluten, and more… The grocery store aisle can be a scary place these days. It seems like there are new stories from social media influencers every day about potent food additives or ingredients that will either kill you or make you live forever. Despite what we hear in the media and find in our Facebook feeds about the dangers that lurk behind the label, the fact is that our food has never been safer than it is today. Why is it then that consumers have never been more worried about the foods they eat? And here's another paradox: At a time when consumers have never known more about nutrition, why is it that obesity is at an all-time high? In November 2018, I took to the TEDx stage in Tysons Corner, Virginia to explore these important topics in my talk, "Why we fear the food we eat."

The rise of "clean eating" and the marketing of "natural" foods has not made us feel safer. Instead, these trends leave us less certain and less confident in the food choices we make. The proliferation of new diets isn't making us healthier; it's just making us more confused.

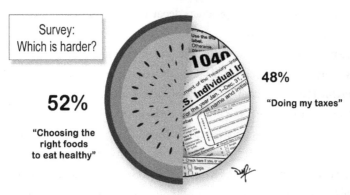

Information source: International Food Information Council Foundation 2019 Food & Health Survey

Making healthy food choices is harder than doing taxes.

According to a survey by the International Food Information Council, a majority of consumers consider making healthy food choices harder than doing their taxes. In an environment like this, what is a consumer to do? How can we sort through all this alarming noise, reduce food anxiety, and make good diet choices that will give us the healthy lifestyle we all want to enjoy?

Information Overload in the Grocery Aisles

It turns out that there are clear psychological principles behind the confusion and fear so many of us are feeling about our food. The way our brains process information has a lot to do with how we respond to food marketing, from the labels on the packages and products on the shelves to the recommendations of social media influencers. We are bombarded with messages and information as we walk the aisles of the local grocery store. Gluten-free, GMO-free, cage-free, pesticide-free…it seems the less a product contains, the more a company can charge for it. Today, the average grocery store carries about 40,000 items, presenting a daunting list of choices for every shopper. There are thousands more new products coming to the shelves soon, and a similar number of failed products departing each year.

The dizzying array of food information in the modern world is too much for one person to handle. We already have overly complex lives just keeping up with installing the latest new operating systems. Having to sort out complicated choices about food can easily feel like too much to manage, and our overworked brains want a way out. Just as students look for shortcuts between classes, our minds look for shortcuts in making decisions. Psychologists refer to the mental shortcuts our brains use as **heuristics** and **cognitive biases**, and these are important concepts in understanding how we make decisions or form opinions.

Mental Shortcuts: Heuristics and Biases

Heuristics are rules of thumb that help us efficiently solve complex problems by ignoring some of the information. Heuristics keep us from going crazy by reducing the load on our mental processors, but they also have their limitations. Mental shortcuts can leave us susceptible to influences that we may not recognize. And sometimes these simplistic rules lead us to bad decisions. A heuristic that results in consistently incorrect decisions ("systematic errors") is called a **cognitive bias**.

Our beliefs and behavior are shaped by these invisible influences. When we are making judgments and decisions about the world around us, we like to think that we are being objective and logical. Unfortunately, biases can trip us up, leading to poor decisions and bad judgments. These powerful forces can even lead us to choices that are at odds with our actual goals, such as nutritional health. We can become our own adversaries when we are guided by influences we don't understand.

Confirmation Bias

Let's take the example of **confirmation bias,** which is the tendency to interpret new evidence as confirmation of our existing beliefs. We seek out information that confirms our beliefs and we ignore or discount information inconsistent with our beliefs because it's easier to entrench more deeply than it is to change our minds. It's easy to see this bias in others, but nearly impossible to convince them of it. It is also remarkably difficult to recognize it in ourselves. That's the nature of heuristics and biases, but by learning about them and facing them head-on, we can learn to perceive them and their effects, reduce their influence, and make our choices more rationally and logically like we wanted to in the first place.

"

> "It is the mark of an educated mind to be able to entertain a thought without accepting it."
>
> —**Aristotle**

Confirmation bias influences many of our food decisions. From the products we buy to the brands we follow, our perceptions, likes, and dislikes are shaped by our existing biases. This makes it difficult for new facts to filter through to our conscious mind and inform our decisions.

> Biases make it difficult for new facts to filter through to our conscious mind and inform our decisions.

With each new fad diet, confirmation bias keeps us believing in the potential of the diet long after the evidence is in that it doesn't work. With every pound we lose, we credit the diet. With each two pounds we gain, we blame ourselves for a lack of willpower. We forget that in order for a diet to work, people need to be able stick to it. We make excuses for the failures of the products or companies we like, but we question the successes of those we don't like.

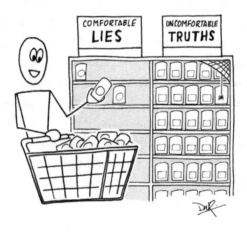

Confirmation bias

From Fear to Enjoyment

In the chapters that follow, I am going to explore how our brains try to make sense of the complex world around us and how it sometimes leads us astray. Confirmation bias is just one example of a misleading heuristic; there are many more. Predispositions can influence the way we perceive brands (such as the "halo effect"), the way we make choices (decision fatigue), and the characteristics of a product we choose to pay attention to (availability bias). Biases like these prevent us from thinking clearly and making accurate decisions, whether the matter at hand is our finances, our health, or the food we choose to eat.

There's no way to avoid all of these potential biases—taking automatic shortcuts is just the way our minds work, after all. But being aware of the biases and shortcomings that are typical of human mental functioning can make a big difference in giving us more rational control over our decision-making processes. My goal is that as you learn how your brain processes information you will fear less, and enjoy more, the food you eat. And this is an achievable goal. We will get there by learning some curious facts about how our minds work, and I'll illustrate them with some interesting stories along the way.

Chapter 2

The Naturalness Bias

When you hear the word "natural," what thoughts or images come to mind? If you think of flowers, puppies, fresh-baked bread, or other wholesome ideas, you're not alone. It's considered a very appealing term.

Do you look for the word "natural" on the food products you buy? A lot of us do nowadays. Consumer demand is pushing retailers to stock more "natural" products on their store shelves, with sales growth outpacing the total food and beverage retail market.

Products that were once only found in "health food stores" or specialty stores like Sprouts Farmers Market, Whole Foods, or Natural Grocers are now available in traditional grocery and convenience stores.

In this chapter we're going to consider the question of what the term "natural food" really means. "Natural" as applied to food is a term that we are apt to use casually. Most of us probably even imagine we could present a reasonable definition of it if asked to do so. But on closer examination, we will find that "natural" turns out to be not such a simple descriptor when it comes to our food.

The Natural Label Sells

The International Food Information Council surveys consumers every year on a variety of topics including how different labels influence their purchasing behavior. According to the 2019 Food & Health Survey, more than a third of consumers were swayed by a "natural" product label when shopping for food, more than those influenced by an "organic" or even a "non-GMO" label.

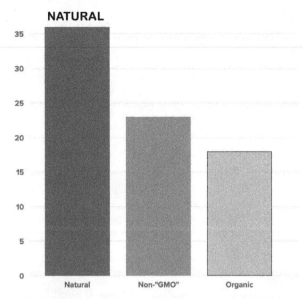

Influence of labels on purchasing behavior: Percentage of consumers swayed by different label types

Information source: International Food Information Council Foundation 2019 Food & Health Survey

The "natural" label is king

Natural Seems Healthier

Words are powerful influencers of behavior. Not only are consumers vastly more likely to purchase a product with the natural label, but they also ascribe a wide range of characteristics to a product bearing such a label. IFIC asked consumers which was healthier, a product with the "all-natural" label or the same product without the label. An astounding 70 percent of consumers surveyed perceived that "natural" products were somewhat or highly likely to be healthier.

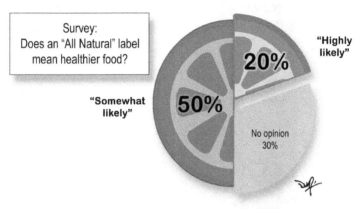

Survey:
Does an "All Natural" label mean healthier food?

"Highly likely"

20%

"Somewhat likely"

50%

No opinion
30%

Information source: International Food Information Council Foundation 2019 Food & Health Survey

Most of us assume "natural" means "healthier.

Clearly consumers believe all-natural food is healthier. But are foods bearing the "all-natural" label really better for us?

It's easy to understand why consumers might think that all-natural products are healthier. Every day we see news stories about pesticides in our food and contamination of our water. We're surrounded by chemicals and highly processed foods that contain many artificial and synthetic ingredients. We worry about the health and safety of our children and we want to do something about it. Eliminating artificial ingredients and synthetic preservatives and colorants seems like a good way to start.

The appeal of the all-natural label has deeper roots in psychology. We have a perfectly reasonable and well-founded fear of tainted products, particularly foods. The Food and Drug and Administration (FDA) was established in 1906 to address the rampant adulteration of food and the food safety issues that resulted.

But the Natural Label Can Be Misleading

The word "natural" clearly has an emotional appeal for consumers, yet most would be surprised to learn that the word itself is not really defined by FDA. The FDA does provide the following policy guidance for food and beverage companies:

> " The FDA has considered the term "natural" to mean that nothing artificial or synthetic (including all color additives regardless of source) has been included in, or has been added to, a food that would not normally be expected to be in that food. However, this policy was not intended to address food production methods, such as the use of pesticides, nor did it explicitly address food processing or manufacturing methods, such as thermal technologies, pasteurization, or irradiation. The FDA also did not consider whether the term "natural" should describe any nutritional or other health benefit. "

—**US Food and Drug Administration**

Since there are no strict criteria for the "natural" label, it can be applied to most packaged foods. And although it doesn't mean nearly as much as people think it does when it appears on a food package, it is a powerful marketing tool.

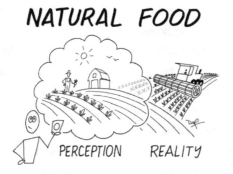

We make many false assumptions about our food based on labels.

Natural Can Be Good or Bad

There are many foods that can kill you, including some mushrooms. The death cap mushroom looks, smells, and tastes delicious, yet as the name suggests, it can be deadly. Other foods, such as almonds, cherry pits, and apple seeds all contain cyanide, which can be lethal if consumed in excess. So while these are "natural" foods, the word "natural" does not guarantee they are safe or healthful.

If some natural foods are good for us and others can kill us, the reality of the term may be more confusing than useful. The IFIC survey found consumers not only believe the "natural" label on a food package implies the food is "healthier," they also attribute all sorts of other positive characteristics to the food that may not exist. Health professionals refer to this phenomenon as creating a "health halo" around the food, which we will discuss in a later chapter.

We Must Look Beyond Labels

The misleading character of the "natural" or "all-natural" label led Consumer Reports to ask the FDA to ban the use of the term on food packages. According to a 2014 survey, that organization found that, "More than 75 percent attribute specific meaning to the word, such as: contains no artificial ingredients, artificial colors, or genetically modified organisms (GMOs). Or for meat and poultry, that the animals were never given antibiotics or artificial growth hormones. None of that is necessarily true."

Our predilection for the word natural has its roots in the "naturalness bias." The naturalness bias is just what it sounds like: it is a preference for products that are labeled as natural. Research has shown that people rate food products (e.g., soda, smoothies, or bean dip) to be healthier and lower in calories when labeled as natural compared to the same type of food without the label, even though calorie content was the same.[7] A "naturalness bias" also appears to have an impact on perceptions of unhealthy behaviors, suggesting that junk food bearing the "natural" label will be perceived more favorably.[8]

The "naturalness bias" leads people to believe that foods with a natural label are both better and safer than foods without that label. The reality, of course, is that anything we consider natural can be good or bad for us, just like the many things that do not come from nature. We must look beyond the naturalness bias to make informed food choices.

Chapter 3

Decision Fatigue

Why do we make bad food choices? One reason is tired brains.

Consider the following scenario: It's seven o'clock in the evening and you make your way through the grocery store aisle, trying to remember the items on the shopping list that you left on the door of the refrigerator. Half the items in your cart weren't on the list, you're pretty sure of that, but it's dinner time and the snacks are looking pretty good. As you check out, you drop a Snickers on the belt. You haven't had one in a long time, so you treat yourself. As you pay the cashier, you vaguely recall…there's a reason you're not supposed to shop for food when you're hungry.

Reflex Decision-Making

Nobody wants to overeat. We all understand that overeating can lead to weight gain, obesity, and chronic diseases, and that we should be thoughtful and deliberate in our choices of what to buy and consume.

Many of us think that the decisions we make are under our control, but the truth is that they often aren't. In the real world of our daily lives, many important decisions are made automatically, or by reflex, without much thought. Too often, these quick decisions actually run counter to our stated goals or deepest desires. We can blame it on our brains.

According to Daniel Kahneman, Nobel Prize laureate and author of *Thinking Fast and Slow*, we have a fast-thinking part of our brain and a slow-thinking part. The fast-thinking part gets us through our days, making gut decisions about most of the choices we have to make. The slow-thinking part does the heavy lifting when it comes to deep consideration and hard decisions. It also does the math. The slow-thinking part is lazy. It won't do the deep thinking unless it has to. It's also easily fatigued. We will come back to these ideas in Part II.

Why Smart People Make Bad Food Choices

Healthy Food Choices Require Careful Thought

Making choices about what to buy and eat may not be as tough as designing nuclear reactors or calculating the flight trajectory of a rocket, but it still takes a mental toll. The human brain gets tired after an intense round of decision-making or after a long day of making choices. When this happens, our brain leans toward whichever option feels easiest—and this is seldom the best choice for our health. The good, healthy choices tend to require thoughtful consideration.

We all have a lot on our minds these days, and we are already overwhelmed with too many choices. Who's going to pick up the kids, drop off the dry cleaning, get the gas, decide on dinner; the list is endless. When it comes to shopping, it's often too difficult to check all the labels and research each product we put in our cart at the grocery store.

If it feels like things are getting harder, it's because they are. And it's not just because our lives have gotten busier (though they have); it's because we are faced with so many more choices today than we ever had in the past.

Food Choices Today Are More Complex Than Ever

In 1980, consumers went into the grocery store and faced no more daunting challenge than whether to buy Prego tomato sauce or Ragu tomato sauce. There weren't too many other options. By the end of the 1980s, things had changed dramatically. Each of those brands was offering a wide array of sauce varieties, from chunky to spicy and everything in between, and on top of this, the number of competitors was beginning to explode. The story was the same for barbeque sauces, salad dressings and dozens of other products. In fact, more than 112,000 new items reached the supermarkets shelves during the

1980s, including many new sizes and flavors of existing products. Considering that the average supermarket stocked fewer than 10,000 items in the '80s, there was also a lot of turnover. Even now, the challenge gets harder every day because the number of options we have is constantly growing (more than 40,000 grocery items today). Dealing with all this is a mental burden that people didn't have to shoulder in the past.

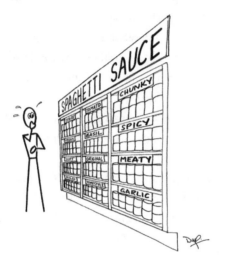

Today's food consumer is overwhelmed with choices.

Online Grocery Shopping Adds Further Distraction

Yet another layer of complexity is added by the popular new wrinkle of online grocery shopping. Most of us are still going to the brick-and-mortar stores to buy our groceries, but online food and beverage sales are rising, and Nielsen Total projects that by 2025, they will hit $143 billion, accounting for a substantial 18 percent of all grocery shopping.[9] There's infinite room on the virtual shelves, which has the potential to really overload consumers already dizzy at the variety available today.

How online shopping will affect the healthiness of our food-buying choices is anybody's guess at this point. Prepackaged guilty snacks are easy to purchase via on-screen icons, whereas healthy vegetables are best selected by hand in person, so online buyers may be more likely to delay their vegetable purchases until they have time to visit the stores themselves.

Our social behavior has fundamentally changed with the advent of the internet, altering the ways that we connect as humans and impacting our herd behaviors in ways that definitely affect our diet choices. Social media floods the online space with information, misinformation, and disinformation, contributing to the decision-making dilemma. We far too often choose our diets because they are popular rather than because they are effective, a point we will return to in Chapter 6, "The Folly of the Crowd."

Tired Brains Make Poor Decisions

According to Deborah Cohen, author of *A Big Fat Crisis: The Hidden Influences Behind the Obesity Epidemic—and How We Can End It,* "We have a limited thinking capacity, so as we use our brains more and more, our ability to think carefully and calculate and analyze is worn down." Even if we don't arrive at the supermarket hungry, we can only spend so much time figuring out what to buy before our brains become overloaded and we begin to make quick decisions based on familiarity or the superficial characteristics of food, notably appearance, convenience, or labels.

Supermarkets are aware of the mental toll that shopping takes, which is why they sell candy and chips at the cash register. Impulse buys mostly happen when our guard is down. Psychologists refer to this phenomenon as *decision fatigue.*

Decision fatigue refers to the deteriorating quality of the decisions we make after a long session of decision-making. The more decisions we make in a row, the worse our judgment becomes.

Decision Fatigue Leads to Unhealthy Food Choices

Having to decide between products with positive and negative characteristics is an energy-draining form of decision-making. A person who is mentally depleted makes very poor choices. Of course, this is exactly what we do when we go shopping for groceries. We make dozens of decisions between fairly similar products. Even when products appear to be identical in terms of nutrition, we still have to compare prices. The price tag tells only part of the story. We also have to check the unit price to be sure which is actually the better buy.

Food choice decision fatigue has further surprising ramifications when we think about how it impacts the rich versus the poor. The less money you have in your pocket, the more time and energy you need to put into every food purchase decision. Rich people don't have to think long and hard about whether to buy the organic or the conventional tomatoes, or Parmigiano Reggiano cheese instead of Kraft parmesan cheese. There really isn't any choice for them to make. As a result, the supermarket induces far more decision fatigue in the poor than in the rich—because each purchase requires more mental trade-offs.

After the mental workout that occurs in the supermarket aisles, it wouldn't be a surprise for someone to pick up that candy bar as they reach the cash register. They no longer have the energy to resist. In fact, by that time, many of us are apt to consider it a reward for the hard work of shopping.

Why Smart People Make Bad Food Choices

Mental Fatigue Also Causes
Unhealthy Food Choices

Decision fatigue is a subset of **mental fatigue**, which can result from decision-making but could be a consequence of hard work or too little sleep as well. Really, anything that depletes our mental reserves can lead to bad decisions. Intuitively, the concept makes good sense, but is there evidence that we can get worn down and make choices we don't really want to make?

It turns out there is quite a bit of research on the topic. In one study, researchers asked people to memorize either a two-digit number or a seven-digit number, and then offered participants either chocolate cake or a healthy fruit salad. The group that had the seven-digit number was much more likely (50 percent) to choose the cake over the fruit salad. It seems that memorizing a bigger number exhausts our mental reserves, making us more likely to give in to an unhealthy food choice impulse.[10]

Similarly, participants in a puzzle-solving study were asked to sit in a room with freshly baked chocolate chip cookies but were told not to eat them. Participants in this group gave up on the puzzle after eight minutes. By contrast, a group allowed to eat the cookies worked on the puzzle for about twenty minutes, about the same as a third group who were assigned to a room without cookies. The thought of the delicious cookies sitting uneaten weighed on the participants, draining their mental energy reserves and ability to work on the puzzle.

In yet another study, researchers showed a group of women an emotional scene from the movie *Terms of Endearment*. Half of them were asked to control their feelings during the scene. The women who were told to suppress their emotions later ate 55 percent more ice cream than the other women![11]

We Often Make Poor Food Choices Unintentionally

"Decision-making, thinking, concentrating, and exerting self-control uses up our mental energy and makes us more vulnerable to choices we wouldn't ordinarily make," Deborah Cohen says.

One of the most troubling aspects of this research is that it suggests that the attention placed on food by the diet industry could be leading to decision fatigue and mental fatigue, which, in turn, result not in healthy food choices, but in loss of control and bad decisions.

We Can Take Back Control

There are a number of strategies you can use to avoid finding yourself in these situations:

- Make important decisions at the start of the day.
- Make strong commitments to prescheduled routines like exercise.
- Make a shopping list and stick to it.
- Don't shop when you're tired or hungry.

Tired brains choose unhealthy foods. Knowing how the brain works gives us power. Certain circumstances are always going to reduce the quality of our decisions, but by planning ahead, we can sidestep much of this trouble, make food choices intentional, and eat a lot healthier in the process.

Chapter 4

The Health Halo Effect

Over the last couple years, late-night revelers who wandered into the nearest White Castle restaurant after closing down a nearby drinking establishment have been confronted with a menu advertising the "Impossible Slider." This is a plant-based burger from Impossible Foods, and it made the jump in 2019 from high-end restaurants with locally sourced ingredients like Founding Farmers in Washington, DC to national chains like White Castle and Burger King.

The year 2019 will likely be remembered as "the year of the meatless burger." Beyond Meat and Impossible Foods achieved significant media attention and reached record numbers of consumers, including many from the meat-eating public. In fact, about 95 percent of people who purchased a plant-based burger this year were meat eaters, according to market research from NPD Group.

With the successful launch of plant-based burgers in Burger King, White Castle, and other fast-food chains, millions of servings of plant-based burgers were purchased that year and even more since then. Livestock producers need not fret quite yet, however. Despite the uptick in interest in plant-based burgers, NPD says that annual consumption of beef burgers remains stable at nearly six and a half billion servings.

But Who Said the Meatless Burger Is Healthier?

Despite the fact that most American adults get plenty of protein in their diet, 61 percent told NPD they want even more protein. Interest in plant-based burgers builds on the years-long trend of consumers searching for higher-protein diets. The meatless burger delivers protein with a perceived plus—according to NPD, many people believe plant-based proteins to be better for you.

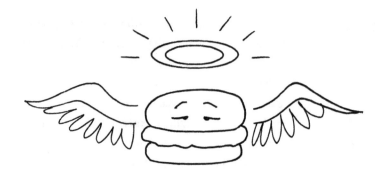

Some of us treat the meatless burger as if it can do no wrong.

A meatless burger sounds like a healthy choice, but is it really? Did the manufacturers even claim that it was healthy, or did we all just assume it? The truth is that the nutritional profile of plant-based burgers is relatively close to beef burgers with respect to dietary concern factors such as sodium, calories, and fat content. It really isn't particularly healthier. Turning to plant-based protein may appeal from an environmental or moral standpoint, but it does not suddenly solve all our diet problems.

One Virtue Doesn't Mean All Virtues

Many consumers today are buying plant-based foods for health reasons, just as consumers have long bought salads because they wanted to make the healthy choice. Unfortunately, our brains often have other plans for us. Good diet decisions are not quite as simple as we'd like them to be. As we discussed in the previous chapter on "decision fatigue," we use mental shortcuts to get through our busy days and make our numerous decisions more efficiently, especially when it comes to food. For example, we may choose a healthy snack such as an apple so that we don't have to worry about counting calories—but the fact is that the apple still has calories. We may virtuously choose the salad rather than a burger—but a salad with dressing may still carry a lot of fat and sugar. When we consider a particular food to be healthy in some respect, our brains all too often completely disregard its other dietary baggage. When it comes to our diets, we tend to treat healthy foods as if they can do no wrong. This is called the "health halo effect," or simply the halo effect. It's another classic mental shortcut that sometimes short-circuits our efforts to build a truly beneficial diet.

The Halo Effect—A Natural Bias

The **halo effect** is, in general, an important type of error in perception that distorts how we see other people, companies, or products. More specifically, "the halo effect is the tendency for positive impressions of a person, company, brand or product in one area to positively influence one's opinion or feelings in other areas."[12] The halo effect helps explain why first impressions are so important. We have all experienced and been influenced by the halo effect at one time or another. When we see a photograph of an attractive person, we tend to ascribe other positive qualities or traits to the person as well, perhaps thinking of them as a good, smart, or successful person. Juries are more likely to go easy on attractive defendants and companies are more likely to hire them.[13] As we discussed in Chapter 2, "The Naturalness Bias," a single word can have a powerful halo effect: We tend to impute positive qualities to food that features the word "natural" in its labeling, even if those qualities are imaginary.

The halo effect comes from our brain wanting things to be nice and simple, so its endless decisions about what to do can be easier. Our brain wants to hurry up and classify things as good or bad, beneficial or harmful. Unless we pay attention, it will take the quickest and easiest way to get there. Our mental autopilot will overlook complicated truth in favor of a reassuring simplification. When this happens, accurate perception gets left behind.

We Simplify the Truth as a Shortcut

When applied to food, the health halo effect refers to the way we overestimate the healthfulness of an item based on a single factor or claim, ignoring other relevant information. This may occur when we see a food labeled as natural, gluten free, or low-fat. For example, studies have shown that consumers sometimes confuse "low-fat" with "low-calorie," which can lead them to overconsume foods labeled low-fat. The low-fat label gives us permission to eat more than we otherwise would because we feel better (or less guilty) about the decision since we assume the food is also low in calories. Research suggests that this tendency is even stronger for those of us trying to watch what we eat.[14] Our overworked brain wants things to be simple, so it equates low-fat with "good," and under the halo effect it then treats the food like it can do no wrong no matter how much of it we consume. The problem is that food companies often substitute sugar for fat in low-fat products to make the food taste better. For example, a twenty-ounce low-fat frozen yogurt could still have up to five-hundred calories. Hardly an ideal tradeoff for those choosing low-fat products as a weight control measure.

Halo Effect Assumptions Mislead Us

Research on the impact of front-of-package labeling of proteins bars also found a significant halo effect connected to the word "protein" on consumer perception of the healthfulness of the product. The presence of "protein" in the name of the product not only influenced perceptions of protein content, but it also increased consumer perceptions of fiber and iron content in the bar—which are totally unrelated dietary concern factors. The presence of a health halo effect was quite clear.[15]

Health halos also influence our judgments about restaurants. If we believe we are eating at a healthy restaurant, we tend to assume *all* the food they serve is healthy. For example, consumers associate Subway with fresh and healthy food, which is how the company positions itself in marketing. By contrast, consumers would not tend to associate McDonald's with healthy food choices. Researchers have found that people buying food at Subway were less accurate at estimating the calorie and sodium content of their meals.[16] The same study found that when people thought they were making healthy meal choices, they were more likely to add toppings, drinks, and desserts, which, in some cases, doubled the calorie count of the meal. This tendency or bias occurred even for consumers who reported that they were trying to make healthy food choices.

Seeing the Truth Beyond the Halo

The virtue of mental shortcuts is that they remove the drudgery of making innumerable decisions each day. The problem, of course, is that many decisions that are made on autopilot should be given more attention because the default choice often is not the best for our health or happiness. Buzzwords like *natural, protein, plant-based* and *organic* are regularly used in food marketing campaigns as key features or selling points of a product because they have a health halo. Such words can fool consumers into thinking that a product is healthier than it really is, which can lead people to make less healthy choices. It is important to remember that a salad smothered in ranch dressing, topped with bacon bits and eggs, may have more calories and fat than the burger you wanted, but didn't buy.

So how do you avoid falling into the health halo trap? Awareness is key. You have to take your mind off autopilot to establish good food choices as your habits. Beware of the halo effect. The "buzz" in buzzwords is intended to distract you from what's important. Remember that what goes on the front of the package is generally the information the food company wants you to know, while the information on the nutrition panel is what FDA and registered dietitian nutritionists want you to know. This includes the recommended serving size for the food. Low in fat could mean high in calories. Low in sodium might mean high in fat. Unless you have an allergy or food intolerance, gluten free usually just means more expensive and less tasty. Instead of allowing healthy-sounding terms to put you at ease, you should think of them as a warning sign to pay extra attention and determine whether the food really will help you build a healthy and beneficial diet.

A Little Attention Will Build Healthier Habits

The moral of the story here is that taking shortcuts is going to cost you one way or another. You make countless food decisions in the course of your life. Most of them are habit-based, made without much thought. Take the time to pay attention and to understand what is really good for you instead of breezing through choices that will have a real impact on your body and your quality of life. Try consulting with a registered dietitian. Once you've identified what is truly best for you, you can turn the autopilot back on and relax in the confidence of having established healthy food-buying habits. You'll be making good choices instead of buying into the appealing, but often misleading halo effect.

Chapter 5

The Dirty Dozen's Dirty Secret

Moms and dads, registered dietitian nutritionists, and doctors all agree that we should eat more fruits and vegetables. They are definitely good for us. The US Department of Agriculture and the Centers for Disease Control and Prevention spend a lot of time, energy, and money trying to convince us to increase our consumption of these healthy foods. Despite their best efforts, however, only about one in ten Americans gets the daily recommended servings of fruits and vegetables.

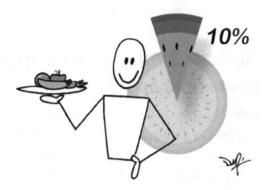

Only one in ten Americans eat the daily recommended servings of healthy fruits and vegetables.

Fruits and Vegetables Can Even Prevent Cancer

The public health consequences of our poor eating habits are significant. According to Teresa Thorne, Executive Director of the Alliance for Food and Farming, "If only half of all Americans increased their fruit and vegetable intake by ONE serving a day, an estimated 20,000 cancers could be prevented every year. Both organic and conventional production methods yield safe and healthy foods that experts everywhere agree we should all eat more of each day."[17]

But Good News Doesn't Get Media Airtime

The scientific consensus in favor of eating more fruits and vegetables doesn't get much airtime on national or local news stations or on social media. Consumers are far more likely to be confronted with news stories about the dangers of pesticide residues on fruits and vegetables. Every year the Environmental Working Group (EWG) issues its infamous "Dirty Dozen" list of the fruits and vegetables with the greatest number of pesticide residues detected.

Pesticide Residue Stories Scare Buyers Away from Fruits and Vegetables

According to the EWG, 70 percent of the produce sold in the US has pesticide residues, including organically produced fruits and vegetables. In 2019, strawberries topped the EWG list for the fourth year in a row. The report states that strawberries are the fresh produce most likely to remain contaminated with pesticide residues, even after being washed, with the dirtiest one containing twenty-three separate pesticides residues.

A number like that is high enough to frighten anybody, and it's no wonder that such stories make consumers leery of buying fruits and vegetables. Nobody wants to expose themselves or especially their children to toxic chemicals, and pesticides would certainly seem to fall into this category. Many pesticides can cause cancer and are highly regulated by the Environmental Protection Agency. It seems to make sense to reduce exposure as much as possible. And yet, tragically, this can result in consumers buying less of the very foods that they most need to become healthier.

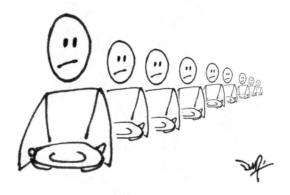

Of the nine out of ten Americans who do not eat their daily recommended servings of fruits and vegetables, how many are missing out because of unfounded fears?

But Our Fruits and Vegetables Are Safe

We need to bear in mind that just because something can cause cancer does not mean that it does cause cancer. As the Swiss physician and philosopher Paracelsus so aptly put it five hundred years ago, "The dose makes the poison." Even water is toxic if we drink too much. Several people actually die each year from its toxic effects—but does that make it a good idea to avoid water? Certainly not! Paracelsus was right: the amount of a material involved makes a tremendous difference in whether it is harmful—or highly beneficial—to human life.

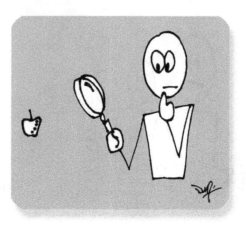

As our food supply becomes safer, we focus on ever smaller concerns.

We are much safer than the EWG Dirty Dozen food pesticide residue list might lead us to believe at first glance. A 2015 analysis of dietary exposure to pesticides in the International Journal of Food Contamination concluded that pesticides in the diet continue to be at levels far below those of health concern. The paper's author, Dr. Carl Winter, Department of Food Science and Technology, University of California, Davis, stated: "Consumers should be encouraged to eat fruits, vegetables and grains and should not fear the low levels of pesticide residues found in such foods."[18]

Notwithstanding good research proving that our food is safe, reports like that from EWG and marketing campaigns by some food producers continue to influence public perceptions about the safety of conventional food compared to food labeled natural or organic. Hundreds of articles are written and news stories presented each year on the purported dangers of pesticides in our food. Consumers are paying attention. But media scare tactics leave consumers afraid rather than informed.

Pesticide Fear Hurts Low-Income Shoppers the Most

Yancui Huang, at the Center for Nutrition Research at the Illinois Institute of Technology, wondered how these types of communications might be impacting fruit and vegetable consumption in populations that cannot purchase organic produce, because of lack of accessibility, budget constraints, or other barriers. Huang and his coauthors conducted a study to see if campaigns like the Dirty Dozen could be discouraging low-income shoppers from purchasing fruits and vegetables.

What he found was that low-income individuals were indeed less likely to purchase any fruits and vegetables after receiving information about the twelve fresh fruits and vegetables with the highest pesticide levels. This is particularly concerning, because, as Huang wrote, "Low-income individuals constitute a financially vulnerable group of people with challenges to meet many daily household needs, including consuming a healthy diet."[19] Stories about the Dirty Dozen and pesticides can be confusing and demotivate shoppers to purchase safe and nutritious fruits and vegetables.

These findings are consistent with the challenges we discussed in Chapter 3's treatment of "decision fatigue," wherein we learned how tired brains make bad food choices. The simple message that "we should eat more fruits and vegetables" becomes more complicated with the news that some produce contains pesticides, which may or may not be a risk to health. Rather than do further research to discover that the pesticide residues on food are perfectly safe, wealthy shoppers simply choose organic produce to reduce their exposure. However, most shoppers are price-sensitive and can't easily opt for higher priced products. When confronted with the need to balance the benefits and risks of conventional versus organic produce for their families, it is often easier to choose neither, and not purchase fruits and vegetables at all. This is a terrible irony, because it means that these consumers are being harmed by information that is supposedly meant to help them.

Pesticide Fear Harms Public Health

There is nothing inherently wrong with sharing information with the public about the presence of pesticide residues in food. Consumers are constantly asking for greater transparency about the food they eat. However, it is also critical to provide consumers with context for such information. Consumers should not be afraid of the food they eat. Instead, they should feel confident that whatever fruits and vegetables they purchase will be safe and nutritious and contribute to the well-being of their family. Our food has never been safer.

Chapter 6

The Folly of the Crowd

Obesity in America has reached epidemic proportions over the last few decades. Obesity lowers life expectancy and increases incidence of serious medical conditions, including diabetes and cancer. Roughly *two-thirds* of all Americans are now overweight or living with obesity, making this a health and food issue of widespread and critical concern.

The Diet Epidemic

The rising prevalence of obesity has led to an accompanying "epidemic," of weight loss *diets*. It seems the more weight we gain, the more diets there are to choose from. Recent data shows that more and more Americans are following (or trying to follow) some form of diet. According to the International Food Information Council, 38 percent of Americans followed a diet in 2019, up slightly from 36 percent in 2018.

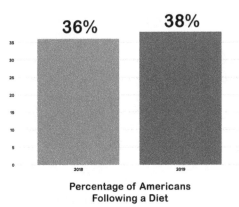

Percentage of Americans Following a Diet

Information source: International Food Information Council Foundation 2019 Food & Health Survey

Diets are a growing trend—just like obesity.

Unfortunately, America's obsession with diets has done nothing to stem the tide of obesity. That may be because many of the diets consumers are following have little support from science. If they don't have scientific validity—and they are not helping people lose weight—why are these diets so popular? That's an important question, and it's what we're going to consider in this chapter.

What Makes Fad Diets So Popular?

New diets can become hot topics more quickly today thanks to their accelerated exposure over the internet, influencing food fashions and shaping product lines in restaurants and groceries across the country. This makes it even easier for more people to jump on the bandwagon. Americans are always on the lookout for the newest diet fad. Remember the Paleo Diet? How about the Keto Diet? Now both are making way for the latest rising star, clean eating.

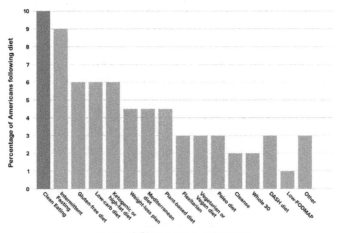

CLEAN EATING

Information source: International Food Information Council Foundation 2019 Food & Health Survey

Clean eating topped the list of popular diets in 2019.

Why Smart People Make Bad Food Choices

Clean eating has been one of the fastest growing diets in recent years. Companies like Panera define *clean eating* as food products free from artificial flavors, preservatives, sweeteners, and colors from artificial sources. While many would describe clean eating as more of a lifestyle than a diet, that has not kept it from becoming the most popular diet of 2019. The clean eating diet was added to the IFIC survey in 2019 and is already the top diet followed by consumers.

Fad Diets Are Popular—But Ineffective

Why is it that consumers jump from diet to diet, following each new craze? One might think that the failure of each new fad diet to deliver the desired health or aesthetic gains would make consumers leery of pursuing the next one, particularly given the substantial amount of money consumers are spending on these diets. But consumer enthusiasm is unabated. The continued growth of the diet industry suggests that the end is nowhere in sight, and American consumers will continue to follow fad diets in large numbers.

We Keep Trying Diets That Don't Work

One reason that individuals tend to follow the crowd, or in this case a fad diet, is because they often turn to people they know as a source of good information. Just like when parents have questions about schools in their area, they typically turn to friends and neighbors for their recommendations. The people we know and trust are who we turn to first when we need information to help us get through our busy lives, even if they don't have expertise in what we want to know. The advantage, however, is that this type of social networking can make decision-making easier.

In Chapter 3, we examined how **decision fatigue** occurs when we're overwhelmed by too many choices. This can lead us to make the easiest decision even when it is not the best choice for us. Given the overwhelming number of popular diets and food fads we're exposed to every day, it wouldn't be surprising to learn consumers often select the diets they are going to follow out of decision fatigue. They simply select what seems to be the most popular diet as a solution to their problems.

And yet, as the stubborn rise of obesity shows, most of the advice provided in the fad diets has not proven effective. Fad diets are simply not solving the problem. Their poor track record ought to leave consumers with very little motivation to follow the next fad diet telling them what and how to eat. So why do consumers fall into what appears to be a deep rut of listening to diet advice again and again from people who obviously haven't a clue as to what will really solve their problems? The answer probably has something to do with **social influence**.

Social Influence Exerts Tremendous Power

The desire to conform to social norms exerts more pressure on our behavior and perception than most of us realize. In 1951, the psychologist Solomon Asch devised an experiment to test the power of social influence. Interestingly, he expected the experiment to show that previous research on social pressure to conform *over*estimated the influence of the majority on an individual's decisions. Boy, was he wrong!

The experimental design included a simple test with an obvious correct answer, which meant that if the subject gave an incorrect answer, it could only be due to group pressure. Fifty male students from Swarthmore College participated in what they thought was a "vision test." Asch put eight people at a time in a room, but only one of them was the actual test subject. The other participants were instructed by Asch and agreed in advance what their responses would be. The real subject believed that the other seven participants were also test subjects like himself.

Each person in the room stated aloud which comparison line (A, B or C in the chart below) was most like the target line. The answer was always obvious. The real subject was positioned so that he sat at the end of the row, and he had to give his answer last.

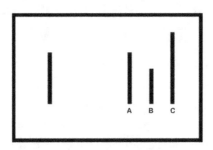

Asch's Experiment chart. Dr. Asch asked, "Which line is most like the first?"

Asch expected that most participants would give the correct answer since the right answer was so obvious. He was sorely mistaken. An astonishing 75 percent of the subjects "conformed" to the influence of the other students at least once and gave a wrong answer. On average, about *one-third* of the test subject answers conformed with the *clearly incorrect* majority. Many people will follow the crowd even when they know the crowd is wrong.

When Asch asked the subjects why they had given the wrong answer, most said that they did not really believe their answers but had gone along with the group for fear of being ridiculed. However, a few said that they really did believe the group's answers must be correct. The study suggests that people conform for two main reasons: because they want to fit in with the group and because they believe the group is better informed than they are.

In the age of social media influencers, it is likely that both forces are at play. Consumers follow influencers on social media because they believe the influencers are better informed than themselves, but they also look to those around them for cues about how they should eat to fit in. They are not necessarily following these cues because they think others are scientifically correct, but rather because they want to be part of the group, and part of fitting in means knowing what and how to eat.

Informed Diet Choices Don't Rely on the Crowd

When it comes to selecting the diet that is right for you, keep in mind that the record shows there is very little wisdom in the crowd. If our goal is to eat healthier, most of us would be better off following the advice of registered dietitians and doctors and avoiding the advice of social media influencers, particularly those with something to sell. And if a family member or friend had success with weight loss, you may want to ask what worked for them, but don't assume it's the right approach for you. On the other hand, if your goal is to be part of the "in-crowd," then the IFIC survey provides a good view of what's hot and what's not.

Next time you find yourself tempted by some new diet craze, ask yourself these questions:

- What is your goal? Quick, short-term weight loss, or a long-term, sustainable reduction?
- Who is promoting the diet you're considering? Family, friends, and popular media? Or registered dietitians (RDs) and registered dietitian nutritionists (RDNs)?
- Is the diet balanced? A balanced diet is a healthy diet.
- Does it encourage exercise? Moving more is always a good idea.
- Does it touch on your mental well-being? More sleep and less stress are a pretty good recipe for good health.

The bottom line is clear: Don't crowd-source your diet wisdom.

Why Smart People Make Bad Food Choices

Chapter 7

Clean Food Fables

In the spring of 2014, Jordan Younger, a "wellness" blogger based in New York City, noticed that her hair was falling out. She was following the "clean" diet she promoted on her Instagram page to her 70,000 followers under the hashtag #EatClean. Younger described herself as a "gluten-free, sugar-free, oil-free, grain-free, legume-free, plant-based raw vegan." She believed she was eating the healthiest of diets. She shared her wisdom through social media and books, and despite Younger not having any qualifications as a nutritionist, her message was popular: 40,000 people bought copies of her twenty-five-dollar, five-day "cleanse" program. Unfortunately for Younger, her dedication to "clean" eating had veered into an obsession, and the diet she was hawking was not improving her health. In fact, as her hair loss visibly attested, the food she ate was actually making her extremely ill. Put another way, the food she avoided could have made her healthy.

Jordan Younger eventually realized her error, "My issue didn't fall into the traditional categories of anorexia, bulimia, or binge eating. Mine was an obsession with healthy, pure, clean foods from the earth, and a fear of anything that might potentially cause my body harm. As it turned out, there was a name for it: orthorexia." In 2015, she wrote a memoir, *Breaking Vegan*, that chronicled her self-destructive fixation with "clean eating" and her obsessive focus on "healthy," "unprocessed" foods. Just because her foods were free from this or that didn't mean that she was eating a healthy diet, and she certainly was not achieving the balance that registered dietitians consistently recommend for good health.

Jordan Younger is not alone; her problem is one we are seeing more often nowadays. Doctors and psychologists warn of a rise in eating disorders linked to taking "healthy" eating to an unhealthy extreme, similar to what happened to Younger.

In this chapter, we will take up the siren song of the food fad.

Clean Eating Is Today's Big Food Trend

As mentioned in the last chapter, clean eating was the most
widely cited diet in 2019, despite the fact it isn't really a diet at all.
Everywhere you look, companies are touting their clean products with
clean labels, and social media influencers are promoting their latest
book to teach you how to eat clean. Powered by social media, clean
eating has been more popular in its reach than any previous school of
nutrition or dieting thought.

Clean Eating Is Hard to Define

So what is clean eating? It means different things to different
people. According to *Clean Eating Magazine*, "The soul of eating
clean is consuming food the way nature delivered it, or as close to
it as possible. It is not a diet; it's a lifestyle approach to food and its
preparation, leading to an improved life—one meal at a time."

Still not clear on what clean eating means?

Panera Bread decided that for them, it was about eliminating
additives. In 2017, Panera announced that it was making its entire
menu of food products free from artificial flavors, preservatives,
sweeteners, and colors as part of its commitment to clean eating and
clean labels. Panera is hardly the only company following this trend.
Companies like Campbell's Soup and PepsiCo have implemented
food transparency through clean labels, and there is a rise in food
start-ups applying clean labels to their new products.

Clean Eating Is Mostly about Fear of Food Additives

Panera's definition of clean eating follows a strong trend. In its 2019 Global Clean Label Consumer Study, ingredient company Ingredion noted that consumers are increasingly looking for products free from additives and artificial ingredients, consistent with the findings in the IFIC survey. The study found that 78 percent of US consumers find it important to recognize the ingredients in the products they buy (an increase from 66 percent in 2011). Interestingly, only about half of consumers consider common ingredients like flour, vegetable oil, and sugar natural. Of course, anything with a chemical-sounding name immediately raises red flags for consumers. Our society has come a long way since we followed the postwar industrial mantra of "better living through chemistry." On the other hand, food fears are not new. A *Peanuts* comic strip from 1966 had the young character Linus deciding he did not want to use a box of chocolate mix after reading on the side that the product was "full of ingredients."

Consumers No Longer Trust Food Companies

Clean eating builds on two separate trends. The first is *transparency*. Consumers want companies to communicate clearly and understandably about what ingredients are in their products. The second is *natural* (with a strong dose of *simplicity*). Consumers want to be able to recognize ingredients and they want as few of them as possible. Companies are catching on, reformulating old products and developing new ones that aim to leverage this trend. For consumers, a "clean label" on a product flags the transparency and simplicity of the ingredient list for the product.

The concept of clean label food products that contain simple and recognizable ingredients reflects a growing desire over the past few years for health-conscious consumers to know what they are putting into their bodies. A survey by the PR agency Ingredient Communications found that as many as 73 percent of consumers will pay a higher retail price for a food product made with ingredients they recognize and trust. The findings underline the growing importance of clean labels and the use of ingredients that are familiar to consumers.

The promise of clean eating is simplicity. Simple foods with ingredients that consumers recognize have the implication that such foods are safer and better for you. While the idea may be simple, the list of foods and ingredients that are forbidden can be quite extensive. In fact, the list is longer than that for most diets.

Clean Eating Demands Clarity— But Isn't Clear Itself

Because there is no specific scientific hook or nutritional basis for clean eating, it is not really clear what foods or ingredients will make the cut. The clean label is more often about consumer perception than it is about anything concrete or tangible. For example, *Clean Eating Magazine*'s definition limits clean foods to those with one or two ingredients. By this definition, virtually none of the foods offered by Panera would qualify. Furthermore, this arbitrary criterion seems to verge toward the same kind of obsessive territory that made Jordan Younger lose her hair. How the number of ingredients in a food is supposed to relate to the healthfulness of the product is never explained.

Clean Eating Is About Demonizing Food Additives

The vocabulary of clean eating, meanwhile, draws on very powerful emotional associations, not on science. Whether we are talking about clean eating, clean labels, or clean energy, the word "clean" has strong psychological connotations. It is synonymous with "good," "pure," "simple," "natural," and "unadulterated." It also brings to mind opposites of these words: "bad," "adulterated," "contaminated," "unnatural," and "processed." In many ways, clean eating is about avoiding bad things. It focuses consumers on fear rather than on the positive attributes of the foods you are allowed to eat. But focusing on fear is what leads to unhealthy diet choices like those of Jordan Younger.

Fear Does Not Lead to Healthy Eating

Limiting ingredients to only those that a consumer recognizes is a dubious basis for nutrition advice. After all, many ingredients in our food today serve an excellent, beneficial purpose, even those that may sound scary. Beyond flavor and nutrition, some ingredients are preventing spoilage or extending shelf life. By improving food safety and reducing food waste, such ingredients are directly contributing to our health and wellness as well as the health of the planet. These are things we should care about.

Unfortunately, influencers and bloggers like Vani Hari, a.k.a. The Food Babe, have made a living—and a financial killing—out of scaring consumers with stories of the chemicals in their food. They capitalize on consumer distrust of Big Food companies and unfamiliar or science-sounding ingredients. They wield words like "chemical" like a hammer, smashing facts and common sense alike. Companies often capitulate in the face of these attacks, irrespective of the safety of the ingredient, and change their ingredients rather than engage in an ongoing public relations nightmare. This is a triumph of fear over good health and sound food production—a tragedy in a world where we should be benefiting from today's easier access to information.

The Clean Truth: Many Food Additives Are Beneficial

Did you know that curry is not a spice? It's a spice mix of five to twenty different spices, which can include things like fenugreek and cardamom. Many scary-sounding words are not only quite natural, but good for you as well. Here are a few more examples of ingredients that are much less alarming than their names seem to suggest.

Pyridoxine

Sounds awful, right? In fact, it is the official scientific or chemical name of vitamin B6, which is an essential nutrient to sustain human life. Pyridoxine is important for protein, fat, and carbohydrate metabolism and for the creation of red blood cells and neurotransmitters. Studies have shown that it may even improve your mood and reduce symptoms of depression.[20]

Ascorbyl palmitate

This is an antioxidant (and a natural compound derived from fat) made from vitamin C and palmitic acid. It is used in foods to prevent spoilage. In your body, it's simply broken down into its parts. Your body uses the vitamin C, and either burns or stores the energy provided by the fat.

Oxidane

If anyone offers you a cup of oxidane, I encourage you to say yes. It is the official chemical name for water. Remember to hydrate.

Eating Healthy Is Not as Simple as Going "Clean"

"Clean" eating may be all the rage, but as with all food fads, it bears thoughtful consideration rather than blind allegiance. The more enthusiastic and determined you are to eat your way to good health, the more mindful you should be about the science behind the trend. Food fads can backfire, as Jordan Younger learned. Don't make your food choices out of fear. If you can't pronounce the ingredients in the food and that worries you, look them up!

Chapter 8

The Snob Effect

If you like good bourbon, you've probably heard of people trying to get their hands on a bottle of the notoriously rare Pappy Van Winkle, produced by the Old Rip Van Winkle Distillery in Franklin County, Kentucky. A few years ago, a friend of mine mentioned he was trying to find a bottle as a gift for one of his clients. While the retail price of Pappy Van Winkle's Family Reserve Bourbon fifteen-year-old is about $120, he expected to pay closer to $700. But there were no bottles available, even at the higher price. Fortunately for my friend, I grew up in Southern Indiana and still had family there. I called my brother, and he called a friend who had a private stash and was willing to part with a bottle at the retail price. Everybody ended up happy. We live in an age of conspicuous production, where the story behind a product is as important as the product itself.

When a product sells in the aftermarket for six times the retail price, a company might be tempted to increase production. But Old Rip Van Winkle Distillery understands the *appeal of scarcity* and knows that increasing supply could kill demand for its product.

There are complex consumer perception issues at work here. The same kinds of factors are playing out in a big way in the world of organic food.

Organic Food Has Gone Mainstream

For decades, organic food sales mostly grew at a double-digit pace, it has reached nearly $50 billion, or about 5 percent of total US food sales, according to the Organic Trade Association (OTA). Organic food is becoming much more affordable and more accessible. Organic's transition from niche to mainstream status was perhaps best exemplified by Amazon's acquisition of Whole Foods in 2017.

One of the first things Amazon CEO Jeff Bezos did when the deal closed was slash prices on a range of organic goods. Fans of organic food celebrated, but the industry has not been quite so thrilled.

Mainstream Status Means No Cachet

By "democratizing" organic food, Amazon's move effectively turned it from a special niche item into a commodity. That shift in consumer perception has had a major effect on sales: The rate of growth in organic food sales has dropped to less than 10 percent during the last few years, hitting just 5.9 percent in 2018, according to the OTA. Rabobank senior analyst Roland Fumasi says, "Organic produce availability has now become mainstream, which means that the organic produce market will continue to more closely resemble the traditionally-grown produce market."

Once a mark of distinction, organic food is now generic and widespread. This is a testament to the past success of organic food producers and marketers, but it also changes how consumers think about organic. The concept of bringing organic food to the masses may have been conceived by people like Alice Waters in Chez Panisse, but it was brought to fruition in the aisles of Walmart. Ultimately, organic food has lost much of the cachet that was driving its high rate of growth.

Cachet Appeal Is the "Snob Effect"

So why is it that just at the moment that organic food has achieved universal awareness and overcome the barrier of cost that had relegated the products to stores like Whole Foods, that growth has slowed rather than soared? Psychologists describe situations in which consumer desire for a product diminishes as its availability increases as the "**snob effect**." The more other people have a product, the less interested new people are in buying it. This is especially true for wealthy individuals, who tend to drop a brand if it goes too mainstream.

Now Plant-Based Is Going Mainstream

What does this mean for other trends? Plant-based foods have seen remarkable growth over the last year. *The Economist* correspondent John Parker declared 2019 was the "Year of the Vegan." A report by UBS bank last year noted, "This has been a breakout year for plant-based meats, with the market growing to just under $5 billion in 2018. The UBS Chief Investment Officer believes this is just the start. With a 28 percent compounded annual growth rate, the plant-based meat market should grow to $85 billion by 2030."

Production constraints for Impossible Foods and Beyond Meat limited expansion in the past, but new facilities appear to have addressed the capacity issues. Today both companies are rapidly signing up new restaurants to distribute their products. Other companies such as Tyson Foods have taken note and are diligently working on competing products. The number of plant-based burger companies is poised to take off. By the end of 2020, hundreds of new plant-based products were on grocery store shelves.

As "plant-based" becomes the fashionable thing to say, we can expect products that have long been made from plants to start adding the "plant-based" label to their products. Peanut butter? That's plant-based. Canned beans? Plant-based. Broccoli? Yep, that's plant-based, too. Look for "plant-based" to become an even more fashionable food label point in the years ahead.

Challenges Ahead for Plant-Based

The biggest threat to the growth of plant-based foods is not competition from beef, pork, and chicken, but competition for shelf space and the consumer's attention. Does anybody truly believe there is a market on store shelves for almost a dozen different plant-burgers? By the end of 2020, many producers of plant-based protein products were already highlighting price, taste, and convenience to break through the noise and win the consumer's attention.

With price competition comes commoditization, and with that the snob effect is apt to kick in. Some of the current appeal of plant-based foods is probably due to its cachet, and as that fades, it will likely slow the growth predicted by UBS. We can expect some product casualties as this plays out, but for the time being, it probably won't be the livestock producers.

The Snob Effect Is Not About Quality

Once you understand the snob effect, you begin to see its influence everywhere. Luxury brands carefully manage their production for this reason. The opportunity to sell a little more product is not worth damage that would be done to the brand's prestige in the long term.

An important point to remember is that the snob effect is not about the quality of a product, but about the social feedback a consumer gets from use of that product. This factor plays into many lifestyle issues involving the products we buy, but food decisions are too important to be made for superficial reasons. Ignore the snob effect and your palate will benefit. Instead of getting annoyed when your favorite artisanal cheese becomes popular and available everywhere, enjoy the chance to eat more of it at reasonable prices. Last year's trends are this year's bargains. Don't resent them. Enjoy them. Look past the snob effect and celebrate the market advances in organic and plant-based foods.

Chapter 9

The Framing Effect

In March 2012, Bettina Siegel, a mother and food blogger in Houston, Texas, sounded an alarm about scary-sounding meat products being served to local schoolchildren. She objected to the use of "lean finely textured beef" (LFTB)—a type of ground beef made from trimmings—in school lunches.[21] She launched an online petition in which she referred to the beef as "pink slime."

Siegel promoted the petition through her "Lunch Tray" blog, asking the US Department of Agriculture to have the "pink slime" banned from school lunches. Social media helped to amplify public concern and opposition to the LFTB. Siegel's local campaign went viral, gaining more than 225,000 signatures in three weeks. The story was picked up by mainstream media, which took it national, then global.[22]

The narrative that emerged, and that drew outrage among the public, was a tale of low-quality food being served to vulnerable children. The "frames" that defined the conversation were quality and health. Within a month, many companies announced that they would no longer use the filler product in their foods.[23]

The Pink Slime Terror Wasn't Really a Terror

LFTB was not actually an unhealthy food and using it reduced costs and prevented food waste, which sound like good things. Why did consumers react with such outrage about this form of beef?

The relentless pursuit of efficiency by food manufacturers has greatly reduced waste from all steps of food processing, but it has not always been appreciated by consumers. Public outrage was unsurprising at the discovery that food companies were feeding

Why Smart People Make Bad Food Choices

consumers food that had previously been thought of as a waste product. Let's face it. Nobody likes to eat trash. And yet, consumers overwhelmingly report a desire to reduce food waste and enhance the sustainability of the food they eat. And they expect companies to do more to deliver these benefits. The problem comes when people don't want to change their eating habits to support such progress.

The Magnitude of Food Waste

According to the United Nations' Food and Agriculture Organization, "roughly one-third of food produced for human consumption is lost or wasted globally, which amounts to about 1.3 billion tons per year."[24] With global population surpassing seven billion—on its way to a projected nine billion or higher by 2050—everyone needs to use the resources available more efficiently. That includes minimizing food waste as much as possible.

Food waste occurs at many points along the supply chain: during harvest, storage, or transportation before reaching the grocery store, at the grocery store, and after the food reaches the consumer. In developing countries, food waste and losses occur mainly "pre-consumer," at early stages of the food value chain and can be traced back to financial, managerial, and technical constraints in harvesting techniques as well as storage and cooling facilities.[25] Food waste in the developed world occurs mostly "post-consumer," when consumers throw away food that has passed the expiration date—even though it is usually perfectly safe to eat. This would rarely occur in the developing world where food is much too precious.

Consumers in many developing countries spend nearly half of their income on food while consumers in the United States spend less than 10 percent.[26]

Was Pink Slime Food Waste or Virtuous Economizing?

An important lesson in the story of pink slime is that how we talk about food matters. Words are powerful, and they can easily evoke emotions and transform public opinion when it comes to the sensitive matter of food. We discussed the effects of the sometimes-misleading term "natural food" in Chapter 2. Characterizing LFTB as waste got it demonized. By focusing the conversation about food waste on sustainability, public attitudes toward food scraps can be modified. In fact, one restaurant was able to convince diners to pay big money for the privilege of eating scraps saved from the rubbish bin. In March 2015, Dan Barber, co-owner and executive chef of Blue Hill and Blue Hill at Stone Barns restaurants, started the pop-up restaurant "wastED" inside Blue Hill's New York City location. The pop-up restaurant exclusively cooked with "food waste."[27] Barber's effort was lauded in articles across the internet for raising the profile, and the bar, on food waste.[28] Nobody seemed to mind they were eating what had previously been considered trash.

The positive response to Barber's project contrasted starkly with the narrative of pink slime back in 2012. The journalist Nara Shin identified the difference in her article "Fine Dining with Food Scraps," saying "WastED is a fine dining experience where taste buds are rewarded with every dish and culinary creativity is showcased. [Barber is] tasking guests with being part of a cultural shift by reframing their own perceptions of waste."[29] As I said, how we talk about food really matters.

It All Depends on the Framing Effect

The frame used to talk about an issue or a product exerts a subtle but significant influence on our behavior, usually without our knowledge. The **framing effect**, as it's called, is a mental shortcut or cognitive bias people use when options are presented in a positive or negative light. The framing as positive or negative affects perception or judgments.[30] Positive framing of products can increase the level of support for or desirability of products and vice versa. We are all familiar with the concept of the glass being half-empty or half-full. On one level, we know that a glass that is half-empty is also half-full. The phrases may mean the same thing. But, on a subconscious level the two phrases also convey significantly different emotions, which can influence our thoughts, our feelings, and our behavior.

A Classic Framing Study

In a famous study conducted by Amos Tversky and Daniel Kahneman, the pioneers of cognitive psychology, participants in an experiment were asked to pick one of two hypothetical treatments for a fatal disease infecting six hundred people. Participants read statements like those below and then selected which treatment option they preferred.

1. Treatment one saves two hundred people.
2. Treatment two has a 33 percent chance of effectiveness for everyone, and a 66 percent chance that everyone dies.

Which option would you pick?

If you're like 72 percent of the people in the original study, you picked option one. Surprisingly, when option one was reframed as four hundred people dying (instead of saving two hundred), only 22 percent of participants were willing to choose that treatment option. Both framings presented participants with the same information—two hundred people would live and four hundred would die either way. The odds didn't change, but the framing did, and it had a dramatic impact on participant perception and willingness to support the treatment. The positive frame won by a heavy margin.

How Framing Sells Cricket Bars

The influence of framing can be seen everywhere in food marketing. Consider the following example of how two insect protein food companies have framed their products.

Grillo is transparent about the nature of the "secret sauce" in its Cricket Energy Bar by proudly placing the word "cricket" front and center on the label. Unfortunately for them, most consumers in the United States have an aversion to eating insects, due to what is commonly referred to as the "yuck factor," that feeling of disgust we get from certain ideas or things. The company attempts to overcome the negative frame resulting from the emphasis on insects as the key ingredient in the food by highlighting the benefits, or positive attributes, of the product, including positive or healthy-sounding words like *energy, organic, chocolate mint, nutrient dense, gluten free, dairy free, paleo* and *future food*.

By contrast, Jungle Bar frames its similar food as an energy bar, a description which has positive associations for most people. The packaging further appeals to our desire for natural foods with simple ingredients. The company doesn't attempt to hide the source of the protein. The phrase "insect powered" is right there, front-of-package. But its placement suggests that it is not vital information, more of an afterthought or a footnote than a bold claim about the contents of the bar. So we don't end up thinking about crickets when we look at this package. Which one would you rather eat? For most Americans, the choice is clear.

Framing Other Plant-Based Foods

Producers of plant-based foods are also well aware of the importance of framing and use the concept to good effect in their marketing. Eat Just foods, manufacturer of Just Egg, which uses mung beans as the key ingredient in its egg-like product, takes an approach similar to Jungle Bar. Rather than try to convince consumers to eat mung bean breakfast sandwiches they frame the product as a plant-based egg substitute. Their product is one of the fastest-selling breakfast sandwiches in the freezer aisle, so consumers seem to agree that describing the product as eggs "made from plants" is more appetizing than "mung bean patties."

Impossible Foods likewise markets its plant-based Impossible Burger without specific reference to just what plants go into its construction.

Future Food Options Will Depend on Good Framing

When we consider the terrible magnitude of food waste in a world where millions of people go to bed hungry every night, we can see that it is going to be increasingly important to frame new alternative food sources in ways that allow consumers to appreciate their benefits rather than recoil from their unconventionality. Negative framing can consign millions of pounds of usable food to the trash bins every day or allow promising products to languish unproduced because they happen to sound unpalatable to current mainstream sensibilities. Tactics like making the reduction of food waste a prominently discussed public virtue or championing the positive impact of an alternative food source could counter negative framing. We have seen in the WastED experiment that clever positive framing can change public opinion completely and make people desire food products one day that they would have thrown out in disgust the day before. A positive frame can change opinion without the need to change minds.

Agricultural engineers and food development researchers are making exciting advances around the globe today, just as food production companies and entrepreneurs are finding innovative new ways to reduce and eliminate food waste at different points in the production chain. The examples cited here illustrate that there are great possibilities ahead—but the spectacle of pink slime reminds us that the role of creative communication and control of the framing effect will be vital if we are to make the most of our potential to feed the burgeoning world. Framing is powerful. It can ruin a good food— or make garbage chic.

Chapter 10

The Availability Bias

The world can seem like a scary and dangerous place these days. We live in the age of anxiety. If you spend too much time on the internet or listening to the news, you might not even want to leave your house at all. According to these sources, there are dangers like air pollution, gun violence, food preservatives, and a hundred other evils lurking around every corner. Our media makes certain that in modern life, we worry a lot about a lot of different things.

But the Facts Are Not So Bad

The Swedish statistician Hans Rosling wrote a book called *Factfulness* with the goal of helping people better understand how to make sense of the daily deluge of information. He felt that with better understanding of the facts, we could all be more hopeful about the future. As a statistician, Rosling spent a lot of time analyzing data about the world around us, and he shared his insights through a number of TED Talks. You can watch an amazing five-minute talk online where Rosling's discussion spans two hundred countries over the course of two hundred years. [31] The positivity in this talk will blow your mind. The trend toward healthier and wealthier citizens is true from Lagos to Bangkok and everywhere in between.

A Great Many Trends Are Positive

A sampling of charts from Rosling's book highlights some of these positive trends, such as the increases in literacy, democratic government, parkland acreage, and food production.

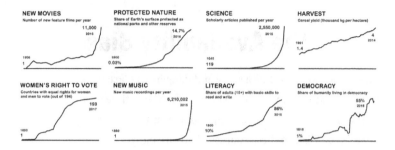

Hans Rosling has charted a great many positive trends in the world today.

Closer examination reveals that even trends like population growth that are widely considered catastrophic are not as bad as most people think. For example, if you had to guess the year when the rate of population growth was the fastest, what might you choose if your options were 1968, 1992, and 2016?

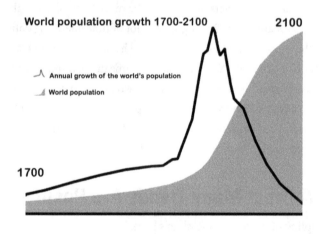

World population growth 1700-2100   **2100**

⋏ Annual growth of the world's population

◢ World population

1700

The population growth rate peaked back in 1968.

The answer is 1968. Since then, the rate of growth has slowed dramatically, and the number of people born each year has pretty much leveled off. The continued growth seen in the accompanying chart is not from a high rate of increase, it's because people are living longer. This is a good news story. By the end of the twenty-first century, the global population will likely begin to decline.

So Why Do We Worry So Much?

If the world is so much better a place today than a hundred years ago, or even fifty years ago, by most measures, why is it that many people, maybe even most people, feel like things are so much worse? The answer to that question can be found in something called **availability bias**, and to illustrate it, let's consider food safety.

Food safety scandals are nothing new. The Food and Drug Administration was created more than a hundred years ago because of a need to confront real and significant dangers to our food supply. Scandals like those of the nineteenth century, such as the swill milk affair of 1850, are rare today, but they cast a longer shadow than ever before. When they do occur, their impact is felt long after the products have been recalled and the perpetrators punished. Why is this?

The Availability Bias

Our brains don't let go of negative stories easily. They hang out in the forefront of our consciousness where our mind can easily access them. This causes old information to color our views and assessments of new situations.

For example, if we read online about an outbreak of a foodborne disease, our brain will go in search of previous examples, and it will latch on to those easiest to recall in order to assess the danger. The bigger an impact an old story had on us, the easier it will be to recall. That usually means the scariest, deadliest, most compelling story… which may or may not be the most relevant.

The more we hear about a story, the easier it is to recall. This is sometimes referred to as "social amplification." In order to save mental "processor time," our brain tends to make judgments about a new story based on its similarity or connection to old news; it is apt to take this shortcut rather than go through the labor of fully processing the new information.

This is an example of a heuristic that researchers Amos Tversky and Daniel Kahneman[32] described as the "**availability bias.**" The availability bias describes how consumers assess the probability of an event with the ease by which occurrences can be brought to mind. This is one of the reasons we worry more about plane crashes than car crashes even though we may realize that car crashes are far more common and kill more people per mile traveled. Plane crashes are vastly less likely to occur to any of us, but they are memorable precisely because they are rare and usually horrific in terms of lives lost. The easy availability of that memory makes that event seem more likely to happen again, or happen to us, even when it is extremely unlikely. That is the availability bias at work, and it can seriously skew our perception of the world around us, especially in an age where negative news events get maximum social amplification online.

Amplified Risks Appear Larger Than They Really Are

Availability bias isn't necessarily bad brain wiring. We are built to remember shocking stories more easily than dull ones so that we will be more sensitive to the possibility of future dangers. The issue arises in modern life when availability bias skews people's ability to judge *probability* or *frequency.*

In order to understand this, let's look at a non-food-related example. Ask yourself—is an American more likely to be killed by a gun-related homicide or radon gas? Most people probably are not even sure what radon gas is, much less that it causes fatalities. It turns out there are more than 30 percent more deaths in the US each year from radon than from gun homicides (21,000 deaths as compared to 15,000). Gun-related deaths, however, get far more media coverage. Media amplification feeds the availability bias, often misleading our perception of risk.

Consider the danger of sharks versus mosquitoes. Which one do you think is the bigger killer? This time, the number of deaths from the two is not even close. By spreading disease, mosquitoes are responsible for hundreds of thousands more deaths each year than sharks.

We Fear What We Do Not Need to Fear

What this adds up to is that we worry about the things people tell us to worry about. How could it be any different? Media networks turn news of scandals into clickbait to increase attention, which is further amplified by our own minds. The result is that we begin to perceive risks where they do not really exist.

Words like "chemical" have become synonymous with toxins. We grow fearful of chemicals and preservatives and food colorings and demand that companies remove them even when—as is the case with preservatives—they are there to make our food safer. We enjoy our food today in a fresh and appealing state even when it has traveled thousands of miles to reach us.

> "The only thing we have to fear is fear itself."
> —Franklin D. Roosevelt

Considering the Facts Can Bring Back Our Confidence

So when you are confronted by the latest news scare, try to remember Hans Rosling's message and "follow the data." Spending a little mental processor time to assess the actual risk to you may produce a very pleasant and comforting revised perspective in the face of an alarmist report. Yes, there are chemicals in the environment, and in our food, and in rare cases, some of it is even hazardous. And yet, despite all that we hear about such dangers, the larger and more important fact is that people continue to live longer and healthier lives. The rate of cancer deaths continues its long, steady decline. People continue to have fewer children, and farmers continue to grow crops with a smaller environmental footprint. This doesn't mean there are no problems. There remain critical global threats like deforestation, greenhouse gas emissions, water pollution, biodiversity loss and, of course, the obesity epidemic. Our past successes should give us hope and strengthen our resolve that we can address the remaining barriers to a nutritious and sustainable future.

Lessons Learned

A Practical Guide

In the foregoing chapters, we have surveyed many of the important cognitive biases that impact the way we think about food. These are some of the biases that most often and most powerfully lead us to make poor food decisions that can undermine our health and the health of our families.

The best inoculation against the harmful effects of such biases is awareness—the raising of which is a large part of the purpose of this book. When we realize how mental shortcuts are short-circuiting our rational decision-making process, we can step in and ensure that our choices are thoughtful rather than accidental. A pattern of deliberate, thoughtful choices leads to good habits, which make the right choices easier. From there, we are well on our way to healthier and happier engagement with food in our lives.

To better enshrine the information we've covered in our memories, I offer the following summary of key biases with reminders about how they play out in our food-related decisions and guidelines to keep your choices for the best.

Confirmation Bias

This is the tendency to hear or seek out new evidence that perfectly confirms our existing beliefs—while remaining deaf and blind to any information that would call for us to change our minds.

- When you stick with a fad diet long after it is clear that it is not actually working for you, confirmation bias is probably making you ignore the evidence telling you to try another path. To counteract confirmation bias, actively seek information from a range of different sources, and try discussing your diet ideas with people who disagree with you, particularly registered dietitians, to see if they might possibly have a point you've missed.

Naturalness Bias

This is the overwhelming tendency to assume that a product is healthier because it is labeled "natural."

- Keep in mind that there are no strict criteria for labeling a food as "natural," and don't give this word too much weight in your food-buying decisions. The "natural" label does not generally convey meaningful information about the nutritional value or the health and safety of a food.

Mental Fatigue

You don't think as clearly and as rationally when you're mentally or physically tired.

- Mental fatigue affects food-related decisions when you select unhealthy snack items on impulse, especially in the checkout lane. Impose a discipline on yourself that says you won't buy unhealthy things unless they are on your grocery list. Don't go shopping for food when you are tired and impulse thinking is on the loose. And never try to "wing" your grocery shopping when you're both tired and hungry at the end of a long day. Always making your grocery list before you get hungry will save you from many sins.

Decision Fatigue

You make worse and worse decisions the more decisions you have to make in a row.

- When you've got too many choices in the grocery aisle and you start to feel lost, that's decision fatigue setting in. Be aware at times like this that your reasoning may not be at its best and avoid deviating from your shopping list until you have obtained good information on new purchases.

Halo Effect

One good quality tends to make us think that a product has other good qualities as well.

- Just because something is "low-fat" doesn't mean it is healthy in any other way. When you see one of these "halo" labels, be on guard for the halo effect and look out for ways in which the product may be sneaking in unhealthy traits behind that golden veil. This is a particularly good time to check the actual sodium, sugar, or other nutrition content, for example, rather than going with your gut.

Snob Effect

I don't want it unless it's hard to get.

- Don't deprive yourself of a good food just because it's gone mainstream and you like to feel special by eating differently from the crowd. We all like to feel special, of course, but buy your food because it's good for you and you enjoy it. Don't let the snob effect make you miss out on something that will enhance your quality of life.

Framing Effect

The context in which we consider an issue can greatly affect the way we end up feeling about it.

- How we frame an issue can have a powerful impact. You might not be tempted by "low-fat vegetarian black bean soup" on a menu, but a bowl of "Cuban black bean soup" sounds pretty exciting. We can harness the framing effect to encourage healthier choices, say getting the kids to eat vegetables. Remember that approaching an issue from a different perspective can dramatically alter the conclusions we reach. Sometimes a disagreement is less about the substance than about the framing.

Availability Bias

The worst stories you hear make you feel like bad things are likely to happen to you, too.

- When you start to become afraid of contaminants in everything you eat because you've heard terrible stories on the internet, that's availability bias misleading you. When you avoid buying fruits and vegetables because you're worried about pesticide residues, availability bias is actively harming you. When you think happy thoughts after reading the word "natural" on a label, that's also the availability bias at work and making you forget that natural things can be bad too. Our food supply is very safe, and we have generally excellent agencies, policies, and procedures keeping it that way. Eat more fruits and vegetables! You will enjoy better nutrition and health and have less stress in your life.

Part II

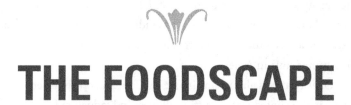

THE FOODSCAPE

Beware Your Foodscape

Part I of this book focused on the *unconscious* biases and invisible influences that affect our food choices. Among these forces we saw, for example, how **health halos** draw us to unhealthy selections with words like *natural, low-fat* and *clean,* and we saw how **decision fatigue** saps our energy and our ability to make smart choices after a long day of tough decisions. We saw how such biases undermine our intention to make choices that promote our own health and that of our families. Part II of the book will consider the myriad *environmental* factors and forces that are also silently influencing the quality and quantity of food we eat. Like the biases mentioned in Part I, these environmental forces are guiding us to make decisions in ways that we are little aware of, choices that directly contribute to the obesity epidemic in America today.

Obesity affects almost one in five children and one in three adults in the United States, putting all these individuals at higher risk for chronic diseases such as diabetes, heart disease, and cancer. It impacts you and me, our parents and children, and our friends and coworkers. All the public health experts, doctors, nutritionists, and diet gurus in the world combined have not been able to reverse this dangerous trend. Furthermore, what once appeared to be a distinctively American public health crisis has now spread to far corners of the world.

Traditional public health campaigns focus on telling people what they should do and how they should eat. Let's face it—such campaigns have been a complete failure: Obesity and its related diseases continue to exceed crisis levels year after year.

Since the early 1990s, government agencies including the Centers for Disease Control and Prevention have been pushing "five a day" initiatives to encourage Americans to consume five daily servings of fruits and vegetables. Thirty years into this effort, only about one in nine Americans eat the recommended servings of fruit. An even smaller fraction, just 9 percent, eat enough vegetables.

Dieting Is Big Business

While the American public's dietary health standard may be on life support, the diet industry is as strong and healthy as ever, with some $66 billion in annual revenue from selling us solutions that by pretty much any measure you care to choose don't appear to be working. The failure of the diet industry has spawned the corporate wellness industry, which offers health and fitness programs and incentives to corporate employees. This has grown into an $8 billion behemoth, also without making much difference in the health of American workers or reducing corporate health care costs.

Bliss Point

Our food environment has changed dramatically since the ancient days of the 1960s. We have exchanged the discipline of regular specific mealtimes for twenty-four-hour access to food and snacks. We have traded the restriction of dining in the kitchen and dining room for the freedom of eating and snacking in every room of the house. In addition, we now include as eating areas the office, the gas station, and pretty much everywhere else we can imagine. We now snack all day long, everywhere we go, at work, in the car, and at home. We snack between meals. We snack in the family room while watching Netflix or Amazon Prime. We snack before bed and other times as well that we probably wouldn't acknowledge. It doesn't fool our bodies that we don't admit these indiscretions to others.

Of course, it's not just when and where we eat that has changed since the sixties. The variety of food options available has exploded in the last fifty years. Do you like Oreo cookies? By some estimates, there are now more than eighty different Oreo varieties and flavors available in different markets around the world. Surely enough to satisfy even the sweetest sweet tooth.

Much has also been written in books—like Michael Moss' 2014 *New York Times* bestseller, *Salt Sugar Fat*—about the many ways food companies manipulate the taste of products to make them irresistible. The companies tweak the recipes, sometimes exploring thousands of variations, looking for the "bliss point"—that perfect balance of sweetness and other flavors and qualities for maximum appeal— which results in maximum addictiveness.

The Shifting Food Environment

From constant snacking to infinite food choices engineered to perfection, we've seen many changes since the 1960s, and today those changes are not just continuing, they are accelerating. The changes go deeper than timing and variety. Everything about our food environment—from the music in restaurants to plate size—has changed. Many of the alterations are much less obvious than the more than eighty types of Oreos in the grocery store and the nonstop snacking, but they are nonetheless significant in their effects. These unperceived changes to the food environment are also having their impact on how we eat.

Some factors in our food environment have less influence over our behavior than we might expect—particularly, sad to say, those factors intended to moderate or improve our consumption habits. For example, we tend to imagine that having more information about our food, such as nutrition facts or recommended serving sizes, should facilitate good decision-making about what or how much to eat. Yet the truth is that these measures do not always have the impact we intend.

Why Smart People Make Bad Food Choices

The Rise of the Foodscape

Food influences are all around us. The food influence environment consists of all the places and spaces around us where we buy and prepare our food, as well as the places where we gather to talk about food. This includes grocery stores, restaurants, food trucks, and our kitchens, but many other places as well, like the blanket or the park bench where we eat our lunch, or even our car as we scarf down a Hot Pocket between meetings, classes, or our kids' sports practices.

These spaces and places containing often hidden influences of food behavior collectively comprise our "foodscape."[33]

Our foodscape is the food environment writ large. Our foodscape has expanded over the decades to include almost every location and moment of our lives. It is not only the kitchen and dining room, but also likely our family room and possibly the bedroom for those who like to snack and watch TV in bed. It may extend to other parts of the house or the backyard where we cook out in the summer. Our local foodscape consists of the food sources within walking distance of our homes as well, which, for me, includes Giant and Safeway grocery stores, a Starbucks, Five Guys, and half a dozen other restaurants as well as the Rite Aid and gas stations that sell snacks and beverages. The broader foodscape extends beyond walking distance to more stores, restaurants, cafeterias, farmers markets, and any other food sources. For our children, the foodscape includes school, but may include the bus, classroom, or school grounds at various times.

The foodscape includes everything that influences our food decisions, so that means our media is part of it too. Food companies, big and small, are vying for our attention. There are commercials on TV and ads online, but also advertising embedded in television programs. It is a shifting context, since a particular space may be part of our food environment one day but not the next.

The foodscape includes overt influences, like the advertising that bombards our senses on TV and the internet, as well as the subtle, covert influences, like the music playing in the background at the local café. It certainly extends to virtual spaces where we turn more and more to make our food-buying decisions. Our appetites are whetted by the food blogs we read and the "food porn" we scroll through on Instagram and Twitter.

Of course, our foodscape also encompasses ourselves—our interior, mental landscape. How our minds lead us to interact with the environment is very important. In that way, everything we covered in Part I of this book is part of the foodscape.

The Big Picture

As we move from the mindscape to the foodscape, we are expanding our view of the influences that are all around us. This helps us look deeper inside ourselves to see how these influences impact our biology and physiology. Understanding the big picture of the foodscapes means understanding the small picture of subtle and hidden influences as well. The way we think impacts what we do and how we behave, but also how we feel.

The foodscape is a wild and sometimes wonderful place. Unfortunately, it is pushing us in many different directions at the same time. Food companies compound the confusion by marketing products rich in refined flours, sugar, salt, and additives that may not be good for us, describing them with terms such as "organic," "local," or "natural" to supply a misleading aura of healthfulness. Our uncertainty is amplified by competing nutritional messages from varied media sources including online and social networks, thought leaders, influencers, and commercial outlets whose messages vary depending on underlying goals, expertise, perspectives, and competing interests. We are, inevitably and understandably, bewildered by these evolving dietary messages.

Past as Prelude

Obesity rates in the 1960s were dramatically lower than they are today. This is not because our parents and grandparents paid more attention to what they ate. They weren't counting calories and they knew nothing about dietary fiber or superfoods. And it certainly wasn't a matter of willpower.

The difference between the past and the present isn't one thing, it is one hundred things, which together make up the foodscape of our current world. If we want to slow and ultimately reverse the tide of health-related illnesses, we need to expand our focus of understanding from the food we eat to the broader food environment. In Part II of this book, we will accordingly examine some of the ways the foodscape contributes to poor food choices and poor health outcomes. Then in Part III, we will explore how the lessons of these unintended influences can support the goal of designing a new, deliberate foodscape that delivers better health outcomes, even without more effort on the part of the consumer. After all, our grandparents weren't nutritionists or dietitians and they somehow managed to get along just fine. They didn't worry about pesticide residues, food additives, ultra-processed foods, or anything else they were putting into their bodies. The foodscape did the work for them. Maybe it can do that work again.

Chapter 11

Eating Fast and Slow

Making healthy food choices seems so easy on the face of it. When I go to a McDonald's restaurant, I have a pretty good idea which foods are healthy and which are bad for me. Even if I wasn't willing to consider a salad, I would know that the triple quarter pounder had more calories than the double, the double more than the single, and the quarter pounder had more than a cheeseburger. Yet somehow, knowing these things in theory and acting on that knowledge in the moment are not the same thing at all.

What is it about how our minds make decisions that leads to so many bad outcomes?

> "What we think of as freewill is largely an illusion: Much of the time, we are simply operating on automatic pilot, and the way we think and act—and how well we think and act on the spur of the moment—are a lot more susceptible to outside influences than we realize."

—**Malcolm Gladwell**, *Blink: The Power of Thinking Without Thinking*[34]

Thinking Fast and Slow

In the 2004 book *Thinking Fast and Slow*, Daniel Kahneman, winner of the 2002 Nobel Prize in economics, explores the many ways our brains lead us astray. As he explains it, our brains have two approaches to decision-making. These two approaches, or systems, as he refers to them, make the decisions that help us get through our days.[35] We are all familiar with these systems, which are really just ways of thinking. What we might call intuition and reason.

We talked about biases and heuristics in Part I of the book. The intuitive system draws on these mental shortcuts, or rules of thumb, which allows for quick decisions. When we have a hunch or feeling about something, that is the intuitive system at work. It is fast. It is efficient. But it doesn't bother too much with nuance or details.

The rational system, by contrast, is methodical and deliberate. You could say it is the part of our brain that "does the math," or heavy mental lifting when needed. The intuitive system generates our first impressions and gut feelings about what we should do. The rational system is that nagging feeling in the back of our mind that second-guesses our initial impression about what to order in the restaurant or buy in the grocery store. It wants to weigh the pros and cons of our decisions to make sure we get the nuances and the details right.

For the most part, these two parts of our brain get along quite well, generally agreeing on the best course of action. But not always.

Unfortunately, decisions about what and how much to eat often put these two parts in opposition to each other. Food choices are notoriously difficult. What we want to eat isn't necessarily the same as what we should eat. And what we should eat depends on what else we've eaten that day as well as our overall health goals. That's a lot to keep track of.

You may have noticed this tension at play the last time someone asked where you wanted to go for lunch. One part of your mind may have been screaming "Five Guys" while another part was prodding you to consider a sandwich from Subway as an alternative. The immediate urge to grab a burger, a bag of fries, and a shake is generated by the fast-thinking, intuitive part of our brains, and this part is biased toward short-term enjoyment. Meanwhile, the part of our brain that is saying, "whoa, whoa, whoa, think about your cholesterol," is the rational, mindful part that considers our long-term health objectives.

Our rational brain brings logical reasoning to bear on the problems it confronts. However, anybody who has struggled with taxes or calorie counting knows that thoughtful deliberation requires effort. Thinking hard is, frankly, tiring, and the more we have to multitask or deal with distractions along the way, the more challenging rational thought becomes. And because problem solving is tiring, our rational brain is lazy. It won't get up off the couch and do math or calculate serving sizes or anything else unless it has to.

Our Lazy Brain

Shakespeare wrote in *Hamlet*, "What a piece of work is a man! How noble in reason, how infinite in faculties." He might have added, "how lazy in practice."

A simple math problem illustrates the limitations of the rational brain. It's called the bat and ball problem. It is a simple problem, so don't let the math part stress you out. Only you will know if you get it right, anyway. Here we go:

A baseball bat and a ball together cost $1.10. The bat costs $1 more than the ball. How much does the ball cost?

What number pops to mind?

Got it?

If your instant answer was 10 cents, I'm sorry to tell you that your intuition, your intuitive brain, failed you.

Don't believe me? Do the math again more slowly. Make sure that rational brain wakes up and gets off the couch to help out.

Once you have taken a minute or two thinking about it, you should see that the ball must cost five cents. Then, if the bat costs $1 more, it must cost $1.05, which, combined with the five cents for the ball, gives you a total of $1.10.

Easy, right? But what happened here? Why do so many of us— about 80 percent in studies—get it wrong?[36]

When we encounter a problem, our brain relies on our intuition to decide if our intuition is sufficient to resolve the issue. The limitations of this approach are obvious, but it is hard to imagine an alternative. If our intuition says, "I've got this," our rational brain can continue dozing on the couch. In the case of the bat and ball problem,

Why Smart People Make Bad Food Choices

our intuition told us that the problem was easier than it in fact was. As a result, it confidently replied with the obvious answer of ten cents, which was wrong.

Our intuition often leads us to be believe it can handle problems that it cannot, so we end up making mistakes. Often, we continue on with our day without even having an inkling that we've made yet another intuition-based mistake. Think about all the decisions we make in the grocery store about what product is the healthiest or which one constitutes the best deal. How often do we stop to really do the math or count the calories? Probably not often enough.

Why do our brains leave us hanging so often? Why did we evolve such lazy brains?

As it turns out, our rational brain is lazy for a reason. It's trying to save energy. There are way too many decisions to make each day in the modern world and, as a result, our brain uses the least amount of energy for each task it can get away with.

Most of the time, when confronted with a choice, intuition takes the lead, and our actions are performed "mindlessly," bypassing rational thought and, many times, even conscious awareness altogether. While we think that our decisions are willful, we are heavily influenced by our environment, as the quotation from Malcolm Gladwell at the start of the chapter notes.

Part II of this book will touch on some of the ways the automatic nature of our intuitive mind leads us astray with the food we eat. Little do we realize that the amount of food we eat is influenced by the size of the portion, plate, or cup. Even seemingly unimportant factors like lighting and music can have a significant impact. Furthermore, repeated behaviors become habits that can then occur without conscious intent.

For the majority of Americans who are overweight or obese, and for the many people around the world suffering a similar fate, the intuitive approach to eating now favors unhealthy options. Our natural tendencies are biased in favor of the sugary snack over the healthy fruit or nuts.

Choosing Healthy Foods Is Hard

Making tough decisions is what people do every day. We want the new iPhone, but we don't really need the new iPhone. Our old phone is perfectly fine. In fact, it's only a year old. While some of us obviously do respect that nagging rational voice in the back of our head, the rest of us give in to temptation and cross our fingers that our spouse will notice the open tab on our computer and surprise us with an early Christmas gift.

Our willpower and the limits of our bank account balance keep our desires in check for the most part. But not, it seems, when it comes to food choices. Why is it that healthy options are so difficult to choose? What makes food unique?

Food decisions are different from most other decisions we make. Food choices tend to force trade-offs between immediate benefits, like a tasty dessert, and future costs. Unhealthy options promise instant gratification and they always deliver. Many potential costs are uncertain and, at any rate, are generally far into the future.

For healthy options, the situation is reversed. The soul-crushing cost of selecting a depressing kale salad lunch is certain and immediate (sorry, kale lovers), but the many splendid, potential health benefits are uncertain and well into the nebulous future. On the other hand, buying a mega bucket of movie popcorn drenched in buttery goodness is guaranteed to enhance my movie-going experience, whereas the weight gain and health problems associated with that bottomless bucket of popcorn are uncertain and far in the future. It's easy to rationalize our overconsumption by telling ourselves that we don't go to movies every day, so we deserve to treat ourselves when we do.

Short-Term Thinking

The holidays are always tough on people trying to lose weight or avoid gaining weight. At Christmastime, my mother places homemade fudge and peanut brittle on every coffee table and countertop throughout the house. Choosing between the immediate joy of my mother's fudge or carrot sticks to tide me over until dinner is easy. The fudge always wins. In the parlance of psychologists, we are "present-biased." We overemphasize immediate costs and benefits, like the jumbo bucket of popcorn at the movies, and undervalue costs and benefits that are delayed, like lower cholesterol from skipping the butter on the popcorn. It's no surprise that this bias results in our favoring unhealthy options, which appeal to intuition.

The future costs of unhealthy eating are not simply far off in time; they are also uncertain. Dietitians sometimes say that there are no unhealthy foods, only unhealthy diets. In other words, any food, including one of my personal favorites, Duck Donuts, can be part of a healthy diet. As a result, the unhealthy foods that we eat carry a real cost only if they are regularly eaten, eaten to excess, or if we fail to go to the gym to work off the extra calories.

So Many Choices, So Little Time

We like to think of our actions or our behaviors as the result of careful thought. But as Kahneman explained through the two-system model for how our brains function, given time, our intentions are generated through thoughtful deliberation, but, more often than not, our actions result from relatively superficial thought processes.

With tens of thousands of products in a typical grocery store and dozens of items on the menu of most restaurants, we are faced with hundreds of food-related decisions each day. Most of us will be hard-pressed to recall even a tiny handful of them. The vast majority of these decisions are made with little conscious deliberation, meaning our intuitive mind is in the driver's seat.[37]

Many food decisions are the result of habits developed from repeated experience. As our actions, decisions, and choices are repeated over time, our brains learn to anticipate the result and our rational brain hands off the matter to our intuitive brain, forming habits. Unfortunately, once our rational brain is out of the picture in decision-making, our actions no longer reflect our intentions. Instead, habits reflect the repetition of past acts that are triggered by the environment.

When it comes to food choices, past behavior is the best predictor of future behavior when habits are involved, whereas our intentions are more relevant when we are engaged in new behaviors. This helps explain why we are able to stick to a new diet for a few days or weeks, but as our rational mind begins to pay less attention to the diet, our intuitive brains kick in and reverts to the bad, old habits that are so ingrained.

While it is possible to form new habits through repetition, our environment remains a reminder or trigger for old behaviors. That's one of the reasons why the eating habits we have at home don't necessarily translate to restaurants and coffee shops. The new environment cues different habits.

In later chapters in Part II of the book, we will examine some of the ways our foodscape influences our habits and behaviors in ways that mostly go unnoticed.

Chapter 12

The SnackWell's Effect

When the Greek physician Hippocrates, known as the father of medicine, intoned, "Let food be thy medicine and medicine be thy food," he was onto something. It has never been clearer that what we eat and how we eat have a tremendous impact on how we look and feel.

Unfortunately, food and nutrition news and information sources are quite noisy today. While some people promote food as medicine, others seemingly believe that most food is poison. The grocery store aisles have become a minefield of big food brands, unpronounceable ingredients, and artificial sweeteners, all of which may or may not be cause for concern.

In Chapter 1, we discussed how most consumers find choosing healthy food more complicated than doing their taxes. We know so much about nutrition that it can be paralyzing.

Not only is it complicated, but nutrition advice also seems to change with the seasons like the latest clothing fashions. I can remember when eggs were part of a healthy and nutritious breakfast. Then we were told to watch our cholesterol, and suddenly egg yolks were off the menu. Egg white omelets took center stage. Recently, the evidence on the nutritional status of eggs has been mostly mixed, so for now, at least, it seems okay to eat them again. Consumers don't really know who to turn to for dependable nutrition advice. As a result, trust is in understandably short supply.

How did we go from simple messages like "eat your vegetables" to calorie counters and micronutrients? When did the simple act of eating get so complicated?

You Scurvy Dog!

Much of what we read about nutrition online or in diet books is of dubious quality and questionable utility. Of course, there is also good nutrition information available as well, based on solid nutrition science. Even the bad information often has a sprinkling of nutrition science behind it. But what is nutrition science, and how did the pursuit of such knowledge contribute to the murky state of the nutrition landscape?

Nutrition science is the study of food and food components and their actions and interactions in relation to disease and health. Our understanding of nutrition science has come a long way over the last fifty years, but the study of the interaction of food and health goes back much further to the most ancient times, as the quote by Hippocrates illustrates. Devastating diet-related diseases such as beriberi and scurvy have virtually disappeared from the United States, though there remain poor communities in the US, and many more overseas, where people continue to suffer from the vitamin deficiencies that cause these diseases.

It is hard to grasp today the suffering once wrought by a disease like scurvy and the fear that for many centuries gripped the men who set off to sea. Scurvy was responsible for millions of deaths of sailors—a deadlier force than storms, shipwrecks, combat, and all other diseases combined. The symptoms are gruesome enough that they do not need to be recounted here, but suffice it to say that sailors feared scurvy above all other threats at sea.

Seventeenth-century ships often set sail with numerous quack treatments for the disease, such as an elixir of vitriol that contained, along with its alcohol, such delightful ingredients as sulfuric acid. The treatments were universally unpleasant, and worse, they were unhelpful at staving off the disease. Some were merely laxatives that surely made matters worse for sailors already suffering from poor nutrition.

James Lind, a Scottish surgeon in the British Royal Navy, is generally credited with demonstrating in 1753 that scurvy can be successfully treated with citrus fruit. The response to the treatment was nothing short of miraculous. Lind not only found a cure, but also demonstrated the ineffectiveness of other treatments of the day, putting many old wives' tales to rest. Or rather, his research *should* have put the matter to rest. Unfortunately, Lind buried the news of his discovery in the middle of his four-hundred-page treatise on the topic of scurvy. As a result, it would be nearly fifty more years, in 1795, before health reformers finally got the memo and persuaded the Royal Navy to give lemon juice to its sailors. It would be much longer still before the connection between citrus fruit and vitamins was discovered, and only then would scurvy be understood as merely the result of a lack of vitamin C.[38]

The War between Sugar and Fat

Less than a hundred years ago, the first vitamin was identified, kicking off a half-century of discoveries tying individual nutrients to nutrition-deficiency diseases. The following decades saw the rise of research on the role of nutrition in more complex diseases, such as cardiovascular disease, diabetes, obesity, and cancers, with the pace of discoveries accelerating in the last two decades.

Sometimes, it seems the more we know, the less we understand. Our current obsession with diets and superfoods and toxic ingredients has its roots in a scientific battle waged in the 1960s and 1970s between scientific luminaries with competing theories regarding the underlying culprit in the rise of certain diseases.

On one side were prominent scientists like Ancel Keys who believed that fat was the major contributor to the growing problem of heart disease. In the other corner, John Yudkin and his compatriots had their sights set on sugar as the key contributor to many diseases, including coronary disease and cancer.

While one may be tempted to acknowledge a role for both fat and sugar in health challenges of the day, every good story must have a villain, and the US Senate needed just that for a report they were writing. Fat ultimately edged out sugar among scientific and policy pundits, and the outcome was embodied in the 1977 US Senate committee report *The Dietary Goals for the United States*, which recommended low-fat, low-cholesterol diets for all.[39]

Of course, the *Dietary Goals* report was merely a skirmish in an ongoing war. In 1980, the US National Academy of Sciences Food and Nutrition Board issued a rebuttal to both sides in the fat versus sugar debate, noting "The recent trend to connect specific dietary habits to disease seems scientifically unsound, and does not take into account the vast variation of nutritional need from one age or life style group to another."[40]

While the National Academy of Sciences may not have put much stock in the ability of the dietary fat and sugar theories to address diseases, scientists continued to develop nutritional models to identify and isolate a single relevant nutrient, assess its isolated physiological effect, and quantify its optimal intake level to prevent disease.

As scientists learned how to break food down into its constituent components, whole foods (not to be confused with Whole Foods) came to be viewed as delivery vehicles for essential nutrients and calories. While this approach seems to make sense, in theory, such reductionist models have not translated well to noncommunicable diseases in practice.

Despite the conclusions of the National Academies report, the 1980 Dietary Guidelines for Americans remained heavily nutrient-focused, recommending that the public avoid too much fat, sugar, and sodium while being sure to eat enough starch and fiber. International dietary guidelines were similarly focused on individual nutrients.

The response from food companies was swift. They pumped out new food products that targeted the recommendations in the guidelines, producing countless options low in fat, saturated fat, and cholesterol and fortified with micronutrients.

Consumers couldn't get enough of products that promised to deliver them from all manner of illnesses. Regrettably, the explosion in these healthy foods did nothing to address the negative trajectory of American health. If anything, it accelerated the trend as obesity continued to soar.

Nutritionist and New York University professor Dr. Marion Nestle summarized it this way: "The problem with nutrient-by-nutrient nutrition science is that it takes the nutrient out of the context of food, the food out of the context of diet, and the diet out of the context of lifestyle."[41]

Rise of the Fad Diet

The failure of the nutrient model to stem the obesity epidemic eventually led to a growing recognition that whole foods were more complex than scientists had imagined. There was also more widespread acknowledgement of the importance of dietary patterns for health and well-being.

In the next phase, it wasn't the food companies that took the lead to exploit the new insights, it was self-help gurus and the social media influencers. They figured out how to package and sell diets, just as the food companies had learned to market nutrients in the 1980s. Food companies were, of course, quick to join in, with a new assortment of products tailored and marketed to the latest diet trends. The diets reflected varying degrees of scientific rigor, from Mediterranean, flexitarian, vegetarian, and vegan to low carb, paleo, and gluten free. Whether you were interested in weight loss, anti-inflammation, or general health, there was a diet plan promoted to meet your needs.

Despite the failure of food-based diet trends to address our weight and health problems, new companies and scientists continue to push the latest research as panaceas for our ills, including prebiotics and probiotics, fermented foods, and gut microbiota; effects of specific fatty acids, flavonoids; not to mention buzzwords like personalized nutrition. Silver bullets abound in the diet food space. We have heard the bold claims often enough that one would imagine that we would become inured against their effects, and yet people are still regularly seduced to give these new products a try. Michael Pollan, noted author of *The Omnivore's Dilemma*, perhaps said it best in a *New York Times* op-ed, "[I]f you're concerned about your health, you should probably avoid food products that make health claims. Why? Because a health claim on a food product is a good indication that it's not really food, and food is what you want to eat."[42]

The Reductionist Manifesto

In the 1980s, we were told to eat more low-fat food and that is exactly what we did. We gorged ourselves on fat-free cookies even though low-fat in no way means zero calories or even low calories. Pollan referred to this as the SnackWell's Phenomenon, named after a popular cookie brand. "By giving a free pass to good nutrients," Pollan explained, "people go there and eat a lot more food. If one SnackWell's is okay because it's low-fat, a whole box is probably better."[43] Pollan observed that consumers or dieters tend to overconsume foods with a health halo, and this came to be known as the SnackWell's Effect.

The obsession with superfoods follows the same pattern as the marketing of foods free from certain nutrients. We are told that superfoods are super because they contain a surfeit of some desirable nutrient. Whether we are avoiding a specific nutrient like sugar, or binging on protein, we are, nevertheless, falling prey to the notion that there is a single fix to our health problems.

The reductionist approach to nutrition has distracted us from the many ways our environment has changed over the last fifty years.

We forget that most people who retired in the 1950s and '60s were not obese. They weren't counting calories or guzzling acai smoothies, either. Neither were they living in fear of pesticide residues on strawberries or trying out the latest Food Babe cleanse.

There is no one thing we can point to that was different back then because everything was different. Consumers back then were not certified nutritionists; they simply had the benefit of a better foodscape.

Over the course of Part II, we will continue to explore ways our foodscape leads to poor nutrition outcomes. This will give us insight into how we might begin to reshape our foodscape to deliver better health results for us all.

Chapter 13

Mind Over Milkshakes

There was a time when nutrition scientists believed that everything we needed to know about weight could be reduced to "calories in, calories out." It seemed so simple. The more we ate, the more we gained. The less we ate, the more we lost. Similarly, our level of activity determined how many calories we burned.

Calories in, calories out, was the conventional wisdom for a long time, but over the last few decades, research has begun to pile up to challenge that simple perspective. Unfortunately, the accounting model was replaced with a not-so-simple collection of views of how our body responds to different nutrients. One size of calorie no longer fits all.

Nowadays, there are plenty of diets available that focus on the kinds of calories or nutrients you eat. Some promote a low-fat diet, others like the Atkins Diet urge you to stay away from carbs, while diets like the Paleo Diet lean on animal protein, nuts, and berries as the key to good health.

Some of these diets grew out of the results of nutrition research, while others had more anthropological roots. For example, according to the Mayo Clinic, the Paleo Diet—also known as the Stone Age, Caveman, or Ancient Diet—is a modern attempt to replicate the diet of humans living from 2.5 million to 10,000 years ago during the Paleolithic age.

While the Paleo Diet may seem reasonably new, it has actually been around for quite a while. It was started in the 1970s by gastroenterologist Walter Voegtlin with the idea that our Paleolithic ancestors could teach us something about how to eat healthy.[44]

These ancient ancestors lived before the advent of agriculture and subsisted on the game they hunted, as well as foods they gathered like eggs, fruits, vegetables, nuts, and roots. The diet was popularized by Dr. S. Boyd Eaton, a professor of anthropology at Emory University,

Why Smart People Make Bad Food Choices

in his 1988 book *The Paleolithic Prescription*. He and his coauthors believed that such a diet is what the human body evolved to eat and that humans were ill-suited to modern diets.[45]

That Pesky Brain

One thing most diet books have in common is the standard emphasis on what you eat. They do not tend to focus on what you think, and they certainly do not dwell on what you think about what you eat. Yet there is a growing body of literature that suggests that the interaction of mind and body is far more influential than we previously imagined.

Now, this doesn't mean that calories don't matter, or that if you can convince yourself that a food doesn't have calories, then you won't gain weight. But it does mean that your body responds differently depending on what it thinks you are eating.

If our minds are influencing our bodies, it raises the question of how the label on a food package may affect the brain, and by extension, the body as well. According to Stanford University professor and psychologist Alia Crum, "Labels are not just labels; they evoke a set of beliefs."

Nearly a decade ago, Crum wondered whether the information conveyed by nutrition labels might be having a physical impact on the body completely separate from the nutritional content of the food itself. As she put it, she wanted to know "whether these labels get under the skin, literally, and actually affect the body's physiological processing of the nutrients that are consumed."[46]

The idea that food labels might cause physical effects grew out of Crum's previous research on the famous "placebo effect," which occurs when our bodies respond as if we had taken a drug even though, in fact, we have only consumed a sugar pill or experienced some other neutral intervention with no expected health impact. There are remarkable examples of the placebo effect in action. In one study, 30 percent of patients given a placebo that they thought was a real chemotherapy drug actually lost their hair—a striking testament to the power of suggestion.

The Mind Is Powerful in Ways that Remain a Mystery

Our expectations about the food we eat play a critical role in determining how we experience food, including our tastes and preferences. Studies of food expectancies suggest an important role for a person's mindset in determining taste and preference. In 2004, professor Samuel McClure, now head of the Decision Neuroscience Lab at Arizona State University, looked at people's preferences for unbranded soda versus the same soda labeled Coke. In the taste test, McClure found that the Coke label had a dramatic effect on subjects' preference.

The effect of brand knowledge for Coke was reflected in brain imaging experiments as well. A Coke lover's brain literally lit up when presented with the Coke label prior to receiving the soda. (Sadly enough, according to brain scans, Pepsi lovers did not experience that same emotional boost when presented with the Pepsi label.) Cultural preferences clearly have a strong influence on expressed preferences.[47]

Study after study has shown that our preferences are strongly influenced by brand information or nutrition labels. McClure's study built on earlier research that found that participants provided with strawberry yogurt or cheese spreads that were labeled "low-fat" enjoyed the products less than they enjoyed the very same products without those labels.[48]

This research is quite distinct from studies discussed in the first part of the book that showed how biases like the halo effect influence what we think of a product. The halo effect leads us to believe that a low-fat product is generally healthier. The studies on preferences show that what we think of a product influences how we perceive or experience a food for better or for worse.

Why Smart People Make Bad Food Choices

Back to Milkshakes

Professor Crum wanted to go one step further than the previous research. She did not want to stop at how the mind experienced labels. She wondered if there was a physiological influence that affected the whole body. More precisely, she designed an experiment to see whether our bodies, not just our minds, would respond to food labels in ways that were inconsistent with the contents or makeup of the food.

To test her theory, Crum whipped up a batch of French vanilla milkshake, which she divided into two smaller batches. This is surely the kind of experiment every college student dreams of signing up for. One batch was put into bottles labeled as a low-calorie drink that she called Sensi-Shake. It was advertised as having 0 percent fat, zero added sugar, and only 140 calories. It already sounds terrible.

The other batch was put into bottles that were labeled as containing an incredibly rich treat called Indulgence. According to the label, Indulgence was everything it purported to be, including packing in enough sugar and fat to deliver a mind blowing 620 calories. I know which study group I would want to be part of.

In truth, both shakes had 300 calories.

Now, we know from earlier research which shake participants should report enjoying more. The Indulgence shake would have been the clear winner. But that was not the question that Crum set out to answer.

Before and after the people in the study drank their shakes, nurses measured participants' levels of a hormone called ghrelin, which is found in the stomach. Ghrelin is sometimes referred to as the hunger hormone. When levels in the stomach rise, that tells the brain that it's time to whip up dinner or find a snack. However, at the same time it is mobilizing the brain to seek out food, it is also slowing down our metabolism on the off-chance there isn't any food to be had.

Whether you find your way to McDonald's for a Quarter Pounder or Chipotle for a rice bowl, you will eventually fill yourself up, be that with fast food or, perhaps, something slightly healthier. When you do, your ghrelin levels will drop. This is the signal, Crum says, that "you've had enough here, and I'm going to start revving up the metabolism so we can burn the calories we've just ingested."

But what if you have a small meal, or a small salad, or a snack? Your ghrelin levels don't drop down that much, and your metabolism doesn't get triggered to ramp up in the same way. Scientists used to think that ghrelin levels fluctuated in response to the nutrients and calories that the ghrelin encountered in the stomach. Consume a big meal and ghrelin responds one way. Snack on a few chips or cookies and ghrelin responds another way.

But that is not what Crum found in her milkshake study. What she found was that the *mindset of indulgence* produced a dramatically steeper decline in ghrelin after consuming the Indulgence shake. Conversely, a *mindset of sensibility* resulted from consumption of the Sensi-Shake, which produced a relatively flat response. Participants' sense of being full or satiety reflected what they *believed* they were consuming rather than the actual nutritional value of what they consumed.

This is a remarkable conclusion. It is not just our minds that can be fooled by labels, but our entire body chemistry or physiology. Our bodies respond not simply to what we eat, but to what we believe we are eating.

Satiety Is a State of Mind

What we think about food is therefore clearly more important than we have been imagining. Our thoughts influence how we perceive food and how we experience it, and they even affect our metabolism as well.

Our brains lead us to enjoy food more (that is, perceive it as better-tasting) if we like a brand, and make us turn up our noses at brands we don't care for. We tell ourselves that we don't like the taste of Coke or Pepsi, but how would we really know? These psychological blind spots are not particularly problematic when it comes to preferences for Pepsi or Coca-Cola, though it may lead us to pay more for brands we perceive as better even if, in an objective sense, they might not be. How do we distinguish our actual preferences from our cultural preferences?

All of these studies taken together paint a pretty bleak picture of our ability to rationally navigate the advertising foodscape that surrounds us.

Of greater concern is our response to foods that are supposed to be healthier for us. If we enjoy low-fat and low-calorie food less because of the label and not because it is inherently worse tasting, then we won't get nearly as much benefit out of these products as we might otherwise. More importantly, if our bodies fail to experience a sense of fullness from eating diet products, then they will leave us hungry again in short order. It is not sufficient that we get enough to eat. We also have to *believe* that we have had enough to eat.

Chapter 14

Supersized Servings: From Popcorn to Coca-Cola

Today we think of 7-Eleven, the home of the Big Gulp, as a marketing juggernaut with its more than 18,000 stores in eighteen countries, but back in the early 1970s, the convenience store chain was struggling to survive. The chain's luck changed, however, in 1976 when Dennis Potts, who was then the merchandise manager for 7-Eleven's stores in Southern California, was approached by Coca-Cola representatives about a new thirty-two-ounce cup design. Potts initially felt that the cups were too big for practical use. The store carried only twelve- and twenty-ounce cups at the time. The Coca-Cola reps offered him two cases for free, so he figured he would find something to do with them.

Potts eventually sent both cases, containing five hundred cups each, to the store with the highest soft drink sales, which was located in Orange County. The most popular item in the store at that time was a sixteen-ounce soft drink bottle that cost fifty cents plus a deposit. The Orange County store introduced the giant Coke cups on a Tuesday for thirty-nine cents. A week later, the store manager called Potts and asked for more of the colossal cups. They had turned out to be anything but impractical. Potts recalled, "We got the message doggone fast. We moved as quickly as we could to get this thing out." The American buyer had responded, and 7-Eleven had a phenomenon on its hands. "It just took off like gangbusters."[49]

Is there anything more American than supersized servings of food? Supersized servings are now a staple of American life, but it has not always been that way. Back in the 1950s and 1960s, American appetites looked pretty much like the rest of the world's. When you bought a cup of Coca-Cola in 1955, it came in a seven-ounce cup.

Why Smart People Make Bad Food Choices

So what happened to set American serving sizes on their epic journey to supersize proportions? Well, it all started with a simple bag of popcorn.

The Popcorn King

In many ways, our current predilection for supersized portions can be traced back to the mad genius of one person. In the 1960s, a man named David Wallerstein had a problem. He needed to increase profits in his movie theaters. Then, as now, movie theaters generated most of their revenue not from ticket sales but from the concession stand. Buttery bags of popcorn, boxes of candy, and soft drinks to wash it all down were a theater's main source of income. As a result, Wallerstein, like other theater owners of the day, spent considerable time and energy looking for ways to increase sales of the high-margin concessions. Wallerstein tried two-for-one deals, matinee specials, and everything else in the marketing playbook, but it wasn't working.

Wallerstein could not get customers to purchase two bags of popcorn or return to the concession counter for a second serving no matter how attractive he made the offers. The deals he tried worked in other industries, but, in the theater, they did not promote concession sales as expected.

Wallerstein eventually wondered exactly where the opposition to these great deals was coming from. Maybe customers were reluctant to purchase a second bag not because they didn't want to eat more popcorn, but instead because they were *embarrassed* to buy a second bag. Perhaps his moviegoers worried that a second bag of popcorn might be seen by others as extravagant, or worse, gluttonous.

Wallerstein eventually hit upon an elegant solution to his problem. Leonard Mlodinow wrote about this epochal insight in his book *Elastic: Flexible Thinking in a Time of Change*, "Wallerstein decided that if he could find a way to circumvent their aversion to buying a second bag, it would help his profitability. It was easy:

just offer a larger bag. And so, Wallerstein introduced a new size of popcorn to the movie-going world: Jumbo. The results astonished him. Not only did popcorn sales immediately shoot upward, but so did the sales of that other high-profit treat, Coca-Cola."[50]

Wallerstein's solution seems breathtakingly obvious today, but back then, it was a revelation. Offering customers larger portions at a slightly higher price worked better than he could possibly have imagined.

At first glance, it might be easy to underrate the fact that all Wallerstein had done was offer popcorn in a larger size. But, by doing so, he had challenged a very basic assumption of marketers of the day. Up until then, the thinking had been that if people wanted to eat more popcorn, they would buy more popcorn, making an additional purchase. But that was not the case at all. The opinions and expectations of others were actually exerting great power over the purchaser in this equation. Outside social forces influence us, and they frequently operate to keep our desires in check. Selling a larger sized bag of popcorn overcame the socially induced inhibition against apparent gluttony. The clever measure solved Wallerstein's concession sales problem but would go on to create tremendous problems for the American diet.

Supersize Nation

I like to think I am a pretty rational person, but at the end of the day, human beings are not very rational creatures at all. In many situations, we don't behave in the way economists predict we should according to rational principles. It never occurred to the marketing gurus of Wallerstein's day to offer larger sizes because they couldn't see how irrational people are. They were stuck in a rational frame of mind and were unable to see what Wallerstein could see—the practical facts of how we as consumers really operate in our socially and emotionally governed world.

According to Mlodinow, "In the 1960s, people viewed consuming larger amounts of food as unattractive, and executives couldn't accept the idea that with their nudging, that might change—that it was simply the act of having to purchase the second helping that stood in the way of unbridled consumption. What's more, many food executives saw larger portion sizes as a form of discounting." At the time, discounting was seen as something that would hurt brand quality, and businesses didn't want to run that risk.

In the 1970s, Wallerstein took a position working for McDonald's, one of the foremost marketing players in the world. Once there, Wallerstein took a page from his movie theater playbook and tried to sell McDonald's CEO Ray Kroc on the idea of selling French fries in larger bags. Business genius that Kroc was, even he did not immediately grasp the significance of Wallerstein's insight. He told Wallerstein that if people wanted more fries, they could simply buy two bags. From Wallerstein's own experience, he knew that this presumption was not true. History would prove him right. McDonald's finally came around to the idea of larger sizes in 1972, and Wallerstein's idea worked again. A special red carboard container designed by a leading industrial designer was devised to present the large size fries as a premium item, and the move was a resounding success.

"It had taken the food industry longer to recognize the law of human gluttony than it took the physics community to embrace the theory of relativity," noted Mlodinow. "In hindsight, the mental adjustment to a framework of thought in which large portions are the standard seems easy." The truth is the transition was not as fast or as easy as we might have imagined.

McDonalds introduced supersized fries in 1992, twenty years after the arrival of 1972's large size. It had taken decades for the new "supersize" paradigm to become the norm, but it had, at last, arrived in all its crispy, salty, savory glory. Marketers were no longer constrained by nutritional needs or even the capacity of our stomachs in what they could offer the consumer. The more they offered, the more we consumed. Nobody seemed concerned that at some point there might be too much of a good thing. How did things get so far out of hand?

The Allure of Value

Looking back again to the 1970s, as the strategy of offering larger sizes was catching fire, consumers everywhere were given the chance to purchase ever-increasing quantities of food for just a few pennies more. For the generations of Americans who had grown up during the Great Depression, larger sizes delivered great value and buyers were delighted to take advantage of such offers.

Value is a great purchase motivator. Who doesn't like to get a good bargain?

My wife and I love to shop at Costco. The enormous containers of mashed potatoes and mac and cheese call out to me. However, I don't want to be eating the same thing every night for a week. We also don't like to waste food, so there is a bit of tension when it comes to bulk food purchases at the warehouse store. Fortunately, there are many deals to be found in the frozen food section as well, so I am always getting my fix of supersized bags at low, low prices. Strangely enough, despite the great prices, we still seem to spend a crazy amount of money on each visit. Good value, it seems, comes at a cost.

The downside for the consumer of supersizing our purchases is much greater in the restaurant than it is in stores like Costco. French fries, soda, and popcorn in restaurants are not the same in their ultimate effect as supersized frozen foods, and certainly not the same as mega-packs of toilet paper and light bulbs. If you buy too much toilet paper, you can stock the cupboards for a rainy day. But diners can't so easily sock away restaurant food until later. When confronted with an oversized meal, most of us just groan as we summon the willpower to finish the last few bites and clean our plate.

There is actually no real value or benefit in eating more food than you want or more than you need. The financial benefit of getting a better value by a few pennies on supersized meals we don't need is nothing compared to the health cost we incur when we consume those excess calories. As America has seen since the '80s, there are dire public health consequences to thinking of extra-large servings of food as "value."

According to Yale University psychologist and obesity expert Kelly Brownell, PhD, in his book *Food Fight: The Inside Story of the Food Industry, America's Obesity Crisis, and What We Can Do About It*, the trend toward large portions demonstrates the convergence of two uniquely American forces: the importance that Americans place on value and marketers' capitalizing on this tendency. It may seem like a deal when a restaurant offers an extra-large serving for a small increase in price, but we all know the company is still making money. After all, McDonald's wouldn't be prodding us to buy the large size if they weren't going to profit from our choice.

The math is actually pretty compelling for businesses selling larger sizes. It may only cost an extra nickel to produce the additional popcorn that goes into a large- versus a medium-sized popcorn, but the vendor may charge the customer thirty-nine cents more for the large size. The vendor reaps a large profit while appearing to offer a great deal.[51] Of course, we generally don't care if the movie theater owner is making money off the large size if we are saving money as well. It seems like a win-win.

The Cost of Supersizing

I can't be the only person who has stood in line at the movie theater concession stand to buy popcorn and done the math only to realize I could get 25 percent more popcorn for an extra quarter. My next thought is, inevitably, that I don't really need the extra popcorn. And then I buy it anyway. My rational brain is too lazy to put up much of a fight. Or maybe it just likes popcorn, too.

Why do we fall for marketing gimmicks? It isn't as if we haven't learned by now how the supersize game works. We all know that we are being tempted to buy more than we want or need by the appearance of a super-good deal.

When we are faced with the question of whether or not to supersize our French fries, it seems like our health should be part of the calculation, but it generally isn't. By the time we are considering what size to purchase, we have already decided we want fries. The decision is not really about health at all at that point. It is about money, and one option seems to provide clearly better value than the other.

Even when the negative health consequences do cross our minds, as they did for me at the concession stand, our brains often talk us into making the unhealthy choice to get the better deal. It's a catch-22. If you buy the popcorn, you feel a little guilty for giving in to supersize marketing. On the other hand, if you don't buy the supersized bucket, you feel like you've missed out on a really good deal. You can easily imagine finishing the small popcorn halfway through the film and wishing you had more.

It makes a crazy kind of sense that if you are going to regret either decision, it's better to be a sucker with a large bucket of popcorn than an idiot with hunger pangs and an empty small bag of popcorn.

My own experience, and doubtless yours as well, suggests that it will not be easy to escape the age of supersized portions through willpower alone. Our brains are suckers for cheap tasty food and good deals, and we like to think about short-term benefits rather than long-term consequences. If we are going to have any chance of reducing the impact of the supersize craze on public health, we will need to find ways of making the healthy decision the *easy* decision.

Fortunately, there are ways to do this. Just as David Wallerstein used a shrewd understanding of human psychology to solve his theater concession problem, we can use our improved knowledge of heuristics and biases to address our public health concerns. We can work with our natural impulses, devising policies and practices that will guide them in directions that are ultimately beneficial. In Part III of this book, we will explore some of the exciting possibilities.

Chapter 15

Plate Tectonics: Shifting Food Portions in America

In February 2003, American filmmaker Morgan Spurlock embarked on a grand experiment, eating only at McDonald's, three meals a day for thirty days. He related the experience in his 2004 documentary *Super Size Me*, describing how he worked his way through every item on the chain's menu at least once over the course of the month. On his epic journey, Spurlock consumed an average of 5,000 calories (equivalent to more than nine Big Macs) every day during the experiment, twice the 2,500 calories recommended for a man his weight.

Spurlock gained twenty-four pounds for his trouble, making for an increase of 13 percent in his body weight in just a month. In addition to the weight gain, he also experienced spikes in his cholesterol as well as mood swings and other negative health outcomes. Spurlock later reported that it took fourteen months after the conclusion of the experiment for him to lose all the weight he had gained.[52]

The More the Merrier

In the last chapter, we talked about the origins of America's love affair with large serving sizes, from movie theater popcorn to supersized fries and sodas, and how things changed from the 1960s to today. We also considered how our love of a good deal leads us to give in to the temptation to purchase bigger sizes.

In this chapter we explore a different, but related question: Why the heck do we eat so much of these monster-sized portions anyway? And I'm not talking here only about extra-large sizes or supersized

Why Smart People Make Bad Food Choices

meals, but large portions in general. We know we shouldn't. We know they are bad for us. But we do it anyway.

It is easy to buy more than we need when we are lured by the notion of a good deal. Value for money is something everyone from bus drivers to bankers understands. But that doesn't explain why we don't save some food for later.

Why don't we take the extra food home more often?

Why do we give in to such obvious temptations when a big plate of food is set before us?

The New Normal

There is nothing more indulgent or exhilarating than the moment your food is served at the Cheesecake Factory. Founded as a Los Angeles bakery in 1972, this international restaurant powerhouse has come a long way in the last fifty years, driven in large measure by the magic of portion sizes.

The serving sizes at the Cheesecake Factory are, in fact, legendary. Whether you order the Ultimate Red Velvet Cake Cheesecake or the Jamaican Black Pepper Shrimp—two of the most popular dishes on the expansive menu of more than two hundred breakfast, lunch, and dinner items—you won't generally be disappointed.

A few years ago, I went to the Cheesecake Factory with my wife and two children for Father's Day. I had experienced the enormous portions in the past, usually gravitating to the jambalaya, but on this occasion, I opted for something different. I ordered the steak, potatoes, and green beans and was prepared to be wowed by the size of the steak and sides.

When the plate landed in front of me, I have to admit to a feeling that bordered on disappointment. The meal seemed lost on the plate. Where were the legendary portions? How was I supposed to eat my way into a calorie-induced coma on this meager bit of beef, I thought?

This was particularly problematic because I had selected the restaurant in large part to teach my children about why it *isn't* always a good thing to clean your plate. Now I was confronted by a meal that looked skimpy, not outlandish. I felt certain I could eat everything on my plate and still have room for a luxurious chocolate peanut butter cheesecake.

Fortunately, I had come prepared. From my wife's purse I pulled out a nine-inch paper plate that we had brought as part of my lesson for the kids. To the horror of my children, I proceeded to replate my food on the paper plate.

To my astonishment it only took half the meal to completely fill the nine-inch plate to overflowing. What was going on here? How could it be that a meal I thought was embarrassingly small was in fact two full meals for an adult?

I turned my attention back to the original plate. I figured I could get away with embarrassing my kids at least one more time—it *was* Father's Day—so I pulled out a tape measure I had brought along for just such an emergency. The Cheesecake Factory dinner plate turned out to be fifteen inches long and twelve inches wide. That means the plate's area was about 25 percent greater than the twelve-inch dinner plate that is the norm in America today, which was more than twice the area of the nine-inch dinner plate I had brought. Now, a nine-inch plate may seem more appropriate for a salad plate than a dinner plate, but that is actually the average dinner plate size from the 1950s. How times change!

If I had not replated the food, I certainly would have eaten more than half the meal, and I was at risk of eating the whole thing. It would not have mattered that I was aware of the Cheesecake Factory's reputation for enormous portion sizes and was on guard to avoid overeating. It would not have mattered that I actually wanted to bring some of the meal home. My brain decided the moment the plate was in front of me that the amount presented was a reasonable amount of food and that I should be able to finish it. Unfortunately, my brain was fooled by the plate size. I would have regretted finishing the meal shortly after taking the last bite, since it takes a while for the brain to receive feedback from the stomach.

The same story of people being served oversized portions is playing out in restaurants around the country every day. However, most people aren't armed with tape measures and smaller plates to protect themselves from their own inclinations.

Bigger Isn't Always Better

The United States is a magnet for tourists from around the world. Some want to experience the wonders of Disney's Magic Kingdom in Orlando, Florida, or the natural beauty of Yellowstone National Park in Wyoming, while others prefer the more grownup pleasures of the Las Vegas Strip. They come for many reasons and to see many things, but visitors from other parts of the world always have at least one common experience. Whether they are supping in the Outback Steakhouse, the Olive Garden, or an all-you-can-eat Chinese buffet, the visitors will discover that serving sizes in American restaurants are, compared to what they know back home, gargantuan. Some visitors might imagine there to be a bit of hype in the stories they have heard from fellow travelers, but then they arrive and find that it isn't an urban legend after all. The Bigfoot of American portion sizes is real. Whether the visitor is arriving from France, Japan, Brazil or Nairobi, the result will be the same: awe at the amount of food they are served and expected to eat.

The large servings are not restricted to restaurants like the Cheesecake Factory, McDonald's, and all-you-can-eat buffets. Big portions are the norm nowadays, even before you supersize them.

Anecdotes might be dismissed in serious analysis, but there is also plenty of hard evidence to back up these impressions. Studies comparing serving sizes at fast-food and other restaurants in the United States and places like France confirm what tourists have known for a long time: The differences are not just in perception, but are, in fact, quite real.[53]

The differences in serving sizes are not limited to restaurants, however. They also extend to portion sizes of packaged goods—and even to the sizes of our homes.

It is tempting to point to cultural differences as the drivers of portion sizes. After all, diners in Paris live in a very different environment than Americans across the ocean. Parisians walk more, and they linger over their meals in ways that might contribute to narrower waistlines. On the other hand, they also consume more butter and fat in their dishes, which generally aren't recommended for those trying to slim down.

Of course, Americans haven't always had a culture that promoted large portions. It is a trend that really took off in earnest in the 1970s, as we've discussed. And other countries are not immune from changing cultural norms or the health consequences that follow from them. The citizens of many countries are now following in the footsteps of Americans when it comes to consumption patterns around serving sizes, with obesity rates skyrocketing even in places like France as a result.

The Joy of Cooking

I'm certainly no master chef, but I do enjoy preparing new dishes. I usually search for recipes using Google but every once in a while, I open a cookbook and look for something exciting, usually something spicy. Paging through a good cookbook is like being a gastronomic tourist on a culinary adventure.

Perfecting a recipe must be hard work, but have you ever wondered how they decide what the correct serving size is for the garlic mashed potatoes or the fettuccini alfredo? The recipes always tell you how many it will serve, but how do the cookbook authors decide what an appropriate serving size is?

Much has been written over the last few decades about expanding portion sizes. We see the increases everywhere we look. Food companies promote the bigger size with "Now 25 percent larger!" on the packages, and fast-food restaurants blanket the internet with ads about big savings on big sizes.

It is not just food companies and restaurants who call attention to portion sizes. You would be hard-pressed to find a restaurant review that didn't mention how big the servings are at a new eatery. Even diet food companies promoting portion control have gotten into the act. You can now buy larger sizes of Lean Cuisine and Weight Watchers frozen dinners.

Increasing portion sizes didn't happen overnight. It required a wholesale revamping of our foodscape, including the pots, pans, and plates we use to prepare and serve our food. University of New York Professor Marion Nestle notes, "Restaurants are using larger dinner plates, bakers are selling larger muffin tins, pizzerias are using larger pans, and fast-food companies are using larger drink and French fry containers."[54]

In one of my favorite studies ever, Nestle and her colleague Professor Lisa Young, also of NYU, dusted off copies of *Joy of Cooking* and other classic cookbooks that spanned more than three decades and sifted through the recipes. They identified 181 recipes for cookies and desserts that appeared in each edition throughout the period. What they found is that while the recipes stayed the same over time, the number of servings one could expect to get from the recipe declined, which meant that the authors expected portions of each dessert to be larger in later editions than they had in earlier editions.

In the 1970s, only a handful of recipes indicated larger portions than previous editions, but by the end of the 1990s, nearly half the portion sizes in the recipes had to be adjusted. The cookbook authors had little choice but to adjust the portion sizes, as consumer expectations about what a typical portion size looked like had changed dramatically. The larger sizes came to be viewed as normal and expected. Restaurants that offered serving sizes typical of the 1960s wouldn't last long in a climate where quantity was synonymous with value. And American appetites knew no bounds.

The New Abnormal

Just how much has changed over the last fifty years is hard to discern when we are only looking at the options on the menus of restaurants today. To really understand how far we have come, we must travel back in time.

Ray Kroc founded the McDonald's Corporation in 1955. At that time, a typical fast-food burger weighed just 3.9 ounces. Now keep in mind, that's not the weight of the hamburger patty, that's the weight of the entire burger, patty, bun, and condiments added together. Today, a typical burger weighs in at 12 ounces, or well over three times the 1955 total. An average order of fries has grown from 2.4 ounces to 6.7 ounces! A large order of fries from McDonalds in 1970 is the same as what you'll get if you ask for a small order today.

It boggles the mind to think about what constituted a normal adult meal back then and what we have come to expect today. Still having trouble imagining how out of hand things have gotten? Consider the fact that a cheeseburger, fries, and milkshake from Five Guys contains nearly 3,000 calories, which is on the upper end of what an adult male would normally consume in a full day.

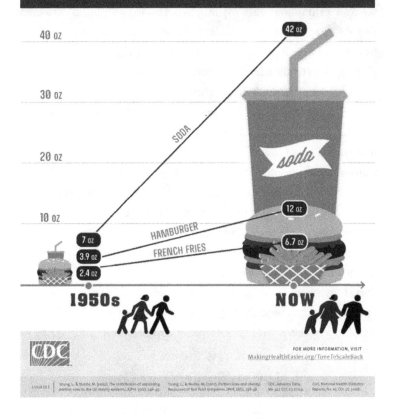

American portions have increased tremendously in size since the 1950s.

Burgers and fries are not the only products that have seen remarkable growth. Cup offerings for soda ballooned from the seven-ounce standard of 1955 to the modern supersize cup, which is nearly six times larger at forty ounces. (That's about twenty-eight teaspoons of sugar if you're keeping track.) Even the kid's menu soda these days is twelve ounces.

We Eat First with Our Eyes

First century Roman gourmand and lover of all things food Marcus Gavius Apicius purportedly observed, "We eat first with our eyes."[55]

I can certainly attest to the impact on my mind and body of seeing a scrumptious dish. My mouth begins to water like a Pavlovian dog as I imagine the first succulent taste of my meal. Before the food has had a chance to dazzle my palate with savory flavors, my mind has already taken the first bite and pronounced judgment over the dish.

Decades of research demonstrate the importance of the visual perception of food on our experience before we take that first bite.

But what about the last bite; what impact do visual cues play on how we feel about that very last bite?

Conventional wisdom suggests that the eyes are also driving the bus when it comes to when we've had enough. After all, the expression, "My eyes are bigger than my stomach," is familiar to everyone who has ever "bitten off more than they can chew." It's not just Americans who are guilty of letting the eyes dictate consumption. In China, they say "yǎn chán dù bǎo" (眼馋肚饱)—envious eyes, belly full—which means pretty much the same thing. Many cultures have their own take on this expression. Perhaps predictably, when given the chance, people everywhere overindulge when it comes to food.

Never Trust Your Gut

Researchers in the 1970s wanted to put this folk wisdom to the test, so they devised an ingenious experiment that involved eating soup from a tube. In order to determine whether it was the stomach or the eyes that decide when we are full, they had to explore eating behavior when the stomach was entirely in charge versus when the eyes were available to influence the amount consumed.

In the experiment, the researchers first determined how much soup each participant would eat under normal circumstances. In this phase, the participants ate the soup from the tube but could track the level of soup in the bowl to see how much they had consumed. The researchers used this as a baseline to determine what a typical serving for each person would be.

In the next phase of the experiment, participants consumed soup from the tube, but were unable to see how much soup was in the bowl. It was left up to the stomach to decide when each participant was full.

The stomach, it turns out, is not a very good judge of how full it is. This is because it takes time for the stomach to realize it is full and send a signal to the brain to put the brakes on consumption. As a result, subjects in the "blind" soup-eating experiment consistently ate more than they had when they were able to see the quantity they had eaten in the bowl.[56]

All You Can Eat

Our eyes aren't always the villain in the story of overconsumption. We use visual cues to determine how much we should eat. We look at a plate of food and we think, "Yeah, I could eat that."

The intuitive mind often thinks it knows more than it really does. Unfortunately, as we learned in Part I of this book, our brain is easily tricked into making bad decisions. People tend to eat more when more food is available. It is as simple as that. We adjust our expectations based on what we are served, and then we eat what's put in front of us.

Don't think this happens to you? You'd be surprised. Many studies have come to this conclusion.

Some lucky participants in a mac and cheese eating study were offered four portion sizes on different days. Researchers found that the bigger the portion size, the more the test subjects ate, on average consuming 30 percent more when served the largest versus the smallest portions. What was particularly telling about this experiment was that participants reported about the same level of satiety or fullness after each meal, with most of the subjects (55 percent) not even noticing that the portion sizes were different each day.[57]

Research in real-world settings confirms the laboratory studies. For example, diners in a restaurant were observed to eat more pasta when larger portions were served. Alas, we all fall prey to the effect of larger portions, and it happens with all types of food, from soup to pasta and from breadsticks to ice cream. We are at least predictable in our gluttony.

A Light in the Darkness

If it isn't just pasta with creamy alfredo or spicy marinara sauce that tempts us to eat more when we are presented with larger portion sizes, then this cloud has a silver lining. The effect can also be exploited to get us to eat more of what's good for us. Experiments have demonstrated that increases in vegetable portion sizes lead to more vegetable consumption when meat and grain portions are kept constant.[58]

The deliberate use of portion sizes to influence eating behavior for healthful physical benefit rather than for ultimately harmful profit points to the foodscape of the future. Such behavioral interventions are invisible influences that work at a subconscious level. They don't require that we be aware of them for them to do their job. In fact, the less we know about them, perhaps, the better. Behavioral interventions in the form of package sizes, portion sizes, and plate sizes can reset what our mind thinks of as appropriate or normal for food consumption.

Half a Sandwich Is Still a Sandwich

The explosive growth in food portions since the 1970s makes portion size an obvious and appropriate target for positive change in our foodscape. However, our tendency to view any serving presented to

Why Smart People Make Bad Food Choices

us as the appropriate portion to consume is not the only cognitive bias at work when it comes to overeating. Research suggests that we are also influenced by the number of items served.

In one study, subjects were offered sandwiches cut to different sizes on four separate days. As with the mac and cheese study, significantly more was eaten when the sandwich portion size was larger. But sandwiches are not the same as a dish like mac and cheese. It's hard to tell how much macaroni and cheese you're consuming when you eat from different sized bowls each day, but most of us know that two half sandwiches equal one sandwich.[59]

In a different study, scientists placed Tootsie Rolls in bowls in a public area of an office. On alternate days there were small or large size candies set out for anyone to take. The weight of available candy was the same each day, but the size of the candy bars, and therefore the number of them, varied. Nobody confuses a full-size Snickers bar with a "fun size" bar. Researchers found that the weight of the candy taken was greater when the unit size was larger. In other words, people tended to take "a serving" whether it was large or small.

The researchers also offered some of the candy in its original size as well as cut in half. Offering half-size Tootsie Rolls halved the amount consumed. As before, the same number of candies were consumed, but the weight of the candy was less.

Office visitors were not confused or misled about the size of the portions. Instead, there was a cognitive bias at work that told them it was appropriate to consume only a particular number of candies, regardless of their size. This is why participants in the first study ate less when presented with plates of sandwiches cut in half. Psychologists refer to this as a "unit bias," which is a perceived appropriate number to eat when presented with a food in a particular form, such as a piece of candy or part of a sandwich. Smaller sizes led to less consumption, even though there was available exactly the same overall amount, and there were no apparent consequences associated with eating more.

Back in the 1960s, David Wallerstein was bumping against unit bias when he was trying to get customers to buy more popcorn and, later, when he went to McDonalds and was trying to get people to eat more fries. He just didn't have a name for it. He imagined people feeling embarrassed at the thought of going back for more, but it turns out that feeling that a single bag was the right amount to eat was a concept even more deeply ingrained than he imagined.

We have an inherent feel or perception of the appropriate number of items to eat of some foods. Wallerstein discovered that larger sizes didn't trigger unit bias and the rest of the world soon followed his lead. Just as larger sizes can lead us to consume more, research also demonstrates the beneficial power smaller unit sizes, in addition to smaller portion sizes, can have on consumption.

Lowball Versus a Highball Glass

I like the idea of being a bartender at a swanky Manhattan bar with dark wood panels on the walls and leather chairs where patrons relax over cocktails and top shelf whiskey during happy hour and then continue the banter and the drinking well into the night. What I don't like about the idea is the thought of memorizing dozens and dozens of different recipes for cocktails. While all of the recipes are readily available in any cocktail manual, searching them up when the bar is packed five deep with people calling out orders sounds like a nightmare.

Then there are the glasses. You also have to remember which drink is served in which glass. Sure, it is safe to say that a martini should come in a martini glass, but some might prefer it in a coupe glass to prevent spillage. And when should you use a highball glass versus a lowball glass?

Bartenders usually don't have degrees in behavioral economics, but they probably deserve them. The combination of cocktail and glass is not chance. The shape of the glass also impacts how we perceive the liquid inside. It is very hard to compare the volume of liquid in a short wide glass, like a lowball glass, to liquid in a tall skinny glass like a highball glass. We overestimate the amount in the tall glass and underestimate the volume in the short glass. Psychologists refer to this as the vertical-horizontal illusion.

When we pour a drink, we use the height of the liquid to estimate how much we've poured. This seems like a reasonable approach, but it doesn't take account of the shape of the glass. Researchers found that when teenagers were asked to pour drinks into short, wide glasses, they poured nearly twice as much compared to when they poured into tall, skinny glasses. Even experienced bartenders poured about 25 percent more into a short, wide glass compared to the amount they poured into a tall, narrow glass.

Once we're aware of the vertical-horizontal illusion, we can see its potential influence everywhere. From the shape of the orange juice cup at the hotel restaurant to the soft drink cup at our favorite eatery, we are being influenced to drink more or less than we imagine. The restaurants may not even recognize the impact their cups and plates are having on us.

Next time you are rummaging through the kitchen cabinet for a glass, give some thought to what you are going to put into the glass. If you are drinking a soda, you might want to opt for a tall, skinny glass. If it's a glass of milk, it may be better to go for the short, wide one.

From Theory to Practice

We can harness these invisible influences in order to bring about beneficial behavioral change that does not rely on conscious individual decision-making like a fad diet does. Just as our brains have been conditioned over half a dozen decades to accept a forty-ounce soda as a reasonable addition to a meal, our brains can be conditioned to view and accept smaller products and portions of unhealthy food and larger portions of healthy ones as the norm.

Behavioral interventions remove the need for willpower from the equation in many situations, thus increasing the chance of achieving our health goals.

We will return to some of these concepts in Part III of the book as we explore methods of reshaping our foodscape to make a healthier lifestyle the default.

Chapter 16

The Limits of Labels

If knowledge is power, then more knowledge must, by definition, make us more powerful, right? Maybe. Maybe not.

I love the smell of coffee. Walking into a Swings Coffee in Washington, DC, I inhale deeply the aroma of freshly ground coffee and exhale a sigh of relief as the day's worries slip away. I step in line to place my order for a flat white coffee and look longingly at the shelves of donuts and brownies, scones and croissants. Most coffee shops have their desserts behind a glass counter so you can see all the tasty morsels to accompany your coffee. Next to the desserts is usually a card telling you how much it's going to cost to satisfy that craving. You may have noticed that nowadays the card also includes calorie information, letting you know how much it is going to set you back, nutritionally speaking, as well.

Whether at a grocery store or a coffee shop, it is hard to argue with the idea of providing nutrition information to consumers about the contents of foods.

The Knowledge Gap

The multi-billion-dollar diet industry is built on the notion that the more we know about the food we eat, the healthier we will be. The whole point of nutrition labels and menu labeling, after all, is to provide consumers with tools to make healthier food choices.

Of course, information and knowledge are not the same thing.

In 1960, very few Americans were obese. It wasn't because people back then were paragons of virtue. They were not watching what they ate and avoiding unhealthy foods. In fact, consumers in the '60s were using lard to fry their chicken and baking with plenty of butter. TV dinners were the rage because they saved time in the kitchen, not because they were healthy options. Consumers back then knew nothing about nutrition.

Things have changed a lot in the last sixty years. Consumers have never known more about health and nutrition than they do today. We know about the dangers of saturated fats and the virtues of omega-3 fatty acids. We have access to low-fat, low-sodium, and low-sugar versions of our favorite foods. We know about the linkages of diet and health. We realize that fatty foods contribute to cardiovascular disease and that carbohydrates with a high glycemic index lead to diabetes. In fact, we are remarkably well-informed about our food and its impacts on our physical health.

And despite all this information, Americans have never been more overweight and obese.

What's going on here?

American waistlines have been expanding for decades. For nearly as long, nutritionists, public health officials, and food policy wonks have advocated for the federal government to do something about it. The dietary guidelines were supposed to inform good food choices, but as we learned in Chapter 12, far from driving better health outcomes, the guidelines kicked off a wave of low-fat, low-sugar, and low-sodium products that muddied the nutritional waters rather than clearing them.

A Brief History of Nutrition Labeling

If you have ever picked up a package of corn flakes, can of cola, or a box of macaroni and cheese, you have seen the FDA-mandated **Nutrition Facts** label, which is prominently displayed on the back of packaged food products in the United States. Although we take the existence of the nutrition facts panel for granted today, not so long ago, it didn't exist.

In November 1990, the Nutrition Labeling and Education Act (NLEA) was signed into law. It was the culmination of years of effort and lobbying by consumer groups. The law had two primary objectives. The first was to provide information on food labels to help consumers make better food choices. The second was to encourage food companies to produce healthier food. Consumer groups hoped that once consumers had a chance to see just how unhealthy many foods were, the food companies would rush to reformulate their products to make them less unhealthy and, perhaps eventually, healthier.

Prior to the NLEA, mandatory information on packaged foods was limited. It seems a bit shocking today, but at that time, nutrition information was required only on foods making a nutrition claim and on those specially enhanced with vitamins, minerals, or protein. The latter requirement explains why all my early memories of nutrition fact panels came from boxes of cereal "fortified with so many essential vitamins and minerals" that I stared at while sitting at the kitchen table having breakfast before school.

The NLEA changed all that and required food packages to contain a detailed, standardized nutrition facts label. This mini placard includes information such as serving size; the number of calories; grams of fat, saturated fat, total carbohydrate, fiber, sugars and protein; milligrams of cholesterol and sodium; and quantities of certain vitamins and minerals. In May of 1994, the nutrition facts label at last made its much-awaited debut in the grocery story aisle.

On January 1, 2020, twenty-five years after the first nutrition facts label appeared on packages, a revised facts panel showed up in grocery stores. Tweaks to the design and information required to be on the package were aimed at enhancing the usability of the label by consumers.[60]

Do Shoppers Read Labels?

So, how often do you read nutrition labels on foods? Do you regularly use them to choose between brands of cereal or energy bars? If you do read labels, what role does the nutrition information play in your food choices? More importantly, do nutrition labels help us make better choices that contribute to improved health?

If you were to ask officials at the Food and Drug Administration whether food labels work, they would probably say yes. Similarly, consumer interest groups often highlight the importance of consumer information in the form of labels. To prove the usefulness of this information, they might point you to FDA surveys of consumer behavior that report that 77 percent of US adults use the nutrition facts label "always, most of the time, or sometimes" when buying a food product. From these results, you might conclude that most people seem to be using nutrition label information at least sometimes. That sounds pretty impressive. And of the people who said they rarely or never use the label, half of them said they did not feel they needed to use the label, which may be because they bought products they were familiar with or that they were satisfied with for their diet or health.[61]

So, if most people are using nutrition labels to make healthy food choices, why is it that so many of us are overweight?

Creatures of Habit

The fact is, that as much as te FDA and consumer advocates would like shoppers to read nutrition labels when making food purchase decisions, the vast majority of shoppers simply ignore nutrition labels altogether.

I asked earlier how often you read nutrition labels. Did you answer always, most of the time or sometimes?

Now try to recall how many nutrition labels you read on your last trip to the grocery store. Did you scan any labels at all? Studies say that the answer is "probably not." This is an area where it turns out we very easily mislead ourselves. Brace yourself for the truth.

Research shows that when we become shoppers, we wildly overestimate how often we use nutrition labels. In one study, researchers found a third of participants claimed to "always" look at calorie content on labels. But when the scientists used eye-tracking technology to check actual behavior, they found that *only 9 percent* really looked at the calorie content. The number of people who looked at information like total fat content and sugar content was even smaller. The truth is dramatically different than what we report.

It's not that the study subjects were intentionally lying to the scientists (though of course, they sometimes do). What we learn from this case is that we are habitually lying to ourselves. We think we look at labels because we see ourselves as the kind of people who look at labels. The truth is, we are creatures of habit. We buy the things we know and like. This means that updating nutritional labels will only have so much impact on those decisions or behaviors. Once again, the lesson is that we don't know ourselves and our brains as well as we think we do.

Do Nutrition Claims Work?

Okay, even if we accept that most shoppers don't read nutrition labels, that doesn't mean that the information isn't helpful to those who do use it, right?

Unfortunately, consumer psychology research doesn't give us much hope here, either. It seems that the more information we give to consumers, the more opportunities there are for them to draw the wrong conclusions and make unhealthy choices.

In Chapter 4, we talked about the halo effect, which leads shoppers to imagine that products with one desirable quality such as "low-fat" also have all sorts of other positive characteristics. Adding more detail to front-of-package claims to avoid misleading claims doesn't help either, since such additions leads many shoppers to experience information overload—aka decision fatigue (remember Chapter 3)—which results in the rational brain tuning out completely. This leaves the intuitive brain in charge of the final decision to buy or not to buy the product, and we all know what happens then. We can see the unhealthy results all around us.

There doesn't appear to be any easy way to win. With simple information, we are open to manipulation by food marketing. With more detailed or complex information, we find it hard to make decisions and we turn to mental shortcuts to help us make a selection, which can also lead to poor choices.

Our Cheating Brains

Sure, making healthy food choices is hard, but we've all managed to make the healthy choice at one time or another. Doesn't this prove that nutrition claims and labels deliver positive results at least sometimes?

Psychologists tell us, "not so fast." The test of good shopping behavior is not whether or not we made one good purchase, but whether the basket of food is becoming healthier overall.

Food decisions are not independent. When we check a label and make the nutritious choice over the tasty but unhealthy option, we feel good about ourselves, like we've won a small battle with obesity. And what do humans always do when they win a battle? They celebrate. This doesn't mean waiting until we get home to open a bottle of wine. Right there in the grocery, we adjust our subsequent purchase or purchases based on earlier purchase decisions. As a result, a shopper who has purchased something healthy is more likely to buy an unhealthy product next.

Psychologists refer to this method of choosing "balancing," "self-licensing," or the "licensing effect." These terms describe the way in which we reward good behavior by being indulgent. When we've done something good, we give ourselves permission to be a little bad as a reward. Our brains, it seems, often have the impulse control of a sixteen-year-old.

So what does this look like in practice? Let's say you walk through the snack aisle at the local grocery store. You want to want to buy the spicy Doritos, but you somehow manage to avoid the salty, tangy temptation and, instead, buy some not-so-yummy, but definitely low-calorie rice cakes. Your brain screams "bland!" Mission accomplished.

Of course, deep inside us, some unconscious judge feels that such a display of mental resolve deserves to be rewarded. The healthy decision will accordingly give you license to buy an indulgent dessert, or something else that is equally unhealthy. This happens because we feel virtuous for the first choice, so we feel we deserve to treat ourselves with the next choice.

This is a huge problem. It is embedded deep in our hardwired psychology, and no nutritional label alone, no matter how improved and informative, is going to have the power to solve it.

Are Nutritional Labels Useless?

FDA and consumer advocates should be realistic about the impacts of labels. If they expect that changes alone will make shoppers choose healthier (read less sugary, salty, fatty) foods, they are likely to be disappointed.

If the conclusions from research about shopper behavior are so grim, what is the use of providing information about added sugars or the calories in more realistic serving sizes on the new labels?

There are two reasons why such information might be useful even if consumers don't use it. First, when a company like Coca-Cola has to explicitly say on its package that a twenty-ounce bottle of Coke contains sixty-five grams of added sugars, or 130 percent of the daily recommended allowance, it might well end up serving as motivation for the company to try really hard to bring these shocking numbers down. And in a competitive environment that values healthy food, there might very well be a "fight to the bottom" among the mega food companies to reduce unhealthy sugars in the products they sell.

The second reason is that even if the label itself fails to have the direct intended effect, *media attention* given to a label change may succeed in having a positive effect on shopper behavior. When a label requirement for trans-fat was introduced by the FDA in 2006, researchers Jeff Niederdeppe and Dominick Frosch found that the news coverage about the change was responsible for reduced sales of trans-fat-laden foods. This occurred even though it was documented that consumers did not fully understand the dangers of eating foods containing trans-fats.[62]

History of Restaurant Menu Labeling

Consumer advocates and public health officials have argued that one of the most straightforward ways of addressing the supersize epidemic is to mandate the labeling of calorie information on restaurant menus. *Menu labeling* seemed like a simple way of giving consumers the information they needed to make smarter food choices. In 2018, the Affordable Care Act mandated menu labeling in all American restaurants, but New York City had gotten there first.

In 2006 New York City became the first major city in the United States to adopt a menu labeling law. It went into effect in 2008. The city required all its restaurants to publish nutrition information about menu items. The rationale was that if consumers had access to nutrition information at the point of purchase and at the moment of consumption, then they would surely make healthier food choices, and the tide of obesity would be reduced.

What a rosy future this new requirement promised! No longer would consumers be swayed by the marketing allure of value meals and supersize options. The menu and calorie information would be there staring them in the face as they chose their food. The negative health impact of those supersized meals would be plain for the world to see in their monstrous, outsized calorie counts. This information, proponents were certain, would guide consumers in their purchasing decisions, leading them to pass on the high-calorie burger in favor of the salad, or skip the supersized fries in favor of the smaller edition. Calorie consumption would decline, and public health would improve.

The presumption of the thoughtful and deliberate proponents of menu labeling was that consumers would be surprised and indeed shocked to learn how many calories were in the beverages and food items offered at their favorite restaurants. Consumers were assumed to be rational creatures who cared deeply about their health. The menu labeling proponents did not take into account the possibility that hungry consumers making decisions at fast-food chain restaurants might care a lot more about convenience, price, and taste than about calories, no matter what the numbers were.[63]

Further diminishing the possible effect of the new regulation was the fact that consumers who cared about calories were already likely to have been well-informed, since calorie information was already available if one cared to look. For consumers who were not well-informed, the direction of the policy's effect would depend on the direction of the surprise about the calorie counts. While some consumers might indeed learn that they were underestimating the calorie content of their favorite menu items, others might actually learn that they were *over*estimating, and might be more indulgent in future purchases. Still others might deliberately seek out the high-calorie items, which might be perceived as a better value than low-calorie alternatives, especially to hard-working laborers or cost-conscious buyers who depend on low-cost calories to sustain them.

About as Well as Expected

George Loewenstein, a behavioral economist at Carnegie Mellon University, did not anticipate big public health improvements as a result of the menu labeling requirement. In an interview with the *New York Times*, he pointed out that it is unclear what impact, if any, menu labeling has on consumer behavior. "There are very few cases where social scientists have documented that giving people information has changed their behavior very much," Loewenstein said. "Changing prices and changing convenience have big impact. Providing information doesn't."[64]

Lowenstein went on to point out that there is a big difference between the upper-middle-class people who promoted menu-labeling policy and the lower-middle-class people whom the policy was aimed at. Getting consumers to understand what the numbers mean is hard enough. Once they do understand, the behavior of consumers from different socioeconomic classes or even different ethnic groups might be quite different. While one group may use the information to inform healthier decisions, others might use it to maximize their calories per dollar. After all, more calories per dollar can sound like good value.

Much Ado about Nothing

Following the implementation of New York City's dramatic menu labeling requirement, a number of studies were conducted to try to answer some of these questions. Interestingly, the studies showed that the posted calorie information did increase the likelihood of customers' reporting having seen nutrition information in the restaurant, reporting using the information, and reporting using it to reduce the number of calories consumed, which all seems like good news. However, the effects all declined over time. And unfortunately, if not very surprisingly from our current perspective, the studies found *no overall impacts* on calories purchased. Not only did calorie information on fast-food restaurant menu boards *not* affect purchases or consumption, but it did not appear to reduce customers' frequency of visiting fast-food restaurants either. Ultimately, the researchers were not able to find *any* consistent change in the nutritional content of foods and beverages purchased at fast-food locations as a result of the regulation.[65] The entire enterprise had been based on a faulty premise and a deeply incorrect understanding of human food psychology.

National Menu Labeling

Despite the general failure of New York's experiment with menu labeling, in May 2018, the US Food and Drug Administration imposed the same policy across America with the national menu labeling provision of the 2010 Affordable Care Act. Like the New York City rule, the FDA law required food chains with twenty or more locations to label their menus with calorie information for all items offered and to post a statement about the recommended total daily calorie intake to provide context for the calorie numbers.

The purpose of the national policy was twofold: first, to increase awareness of the calorie content of foods offered at chain food establishments, which was often underestimated, and second, to encourage restaurants to offer lower-calorie items. The ultimate goal of the policy, of course, was to reduce obesity and its costly related chronic diseases.

Studies examining the outcomes of the national menu labeling requirement found little impact on calorie intake, echoing the findings on New York City's policy. While there was a slight decrease in calories consumed at fast-food restaurants immediately following implementation of the labeling rule, this initial decrease slowly disappeared over the course of just a single year as consumers returned to the previous habits.[66]

The Limits of Labels

The failure of nutrition facts and menu labels to address the obesity epidemic is not a reason to give up on such interventions. Many countries are exploring new approaches that rely on insights into consumer behavior as they try to design new front-of-package labels that may be more effective. And there are other completely different ways of addressing these problems that avoid scolding labels entirely, as we'll see when we talk about environmental solutions.

The challenge of devising effective food labels is made more difficult by the fact that we now realize that many people simply don't want to have more information, especially in certain circumstances. In Cass Sunstein's book *Too Much Information*, he recounts a story from the time he was working for the Obama Administration and had just overseen the publication of the rules for menu labeling. He sent a note to a friend, excited by the prospect of giving consumers this new tool to make healthier food choices. The menu labeling requirement applied to restaurants as well as other businesses like movie theaters.

The friend wrote back, "CASS RUINED POPCORN!" Sunstein immediately understood her point. People go to movie theaters for fun. They don't want to have to think about how unhealthy the popcorn is as the lights drop and the movie begins.

When it comes to information and how we devise our food policies, it is better to live in the world of facts, results, and truth rather than in the world of wishes, intentions, and illusions. Transparency makes good decisions possible, but it is obviously not enough. And clear-eyed, realistic thinking on these matters is desperately called for by the alarming state of our public health. We cannot go on repeating past failures. We need approaches that recognize the ways that food decisions are made by real human beings, not imaginary creatures more rational and responsible than we are in real life. In Part III, we will explore some ways to get our environment working for us.

Chapter 17

Invisible Influences at the Dinner Table

In 1993 as Christmas approached, I was studying law in Paris. My limited funds meant a return to the US for the holidays was out of the question, so I caught a train and then a ferry to England to visit my friends Andi and Vera, who lived in Horsham, south of London. Andi and I shared a passion for spicy food, so the two of us set off one night for a nearby Indian restaurant.

Nearly thirty years later, I can still recall the spicy heat of the lamb vindaloo and the beads of sweat on my forehead as I ate the last bite. But what I remember even more vividly was how full Andi and I were. We practically staggered from that restaurant to the pub around the corner. In fact, we were so stuffed that when our pints of Guinness arrived, neither of us could find room in our stomachs for even a sip of the excellent beer. For the longest time, we both sat at the bar and gazed longingly at our pints. Fortunately, we were patient, and eventually we two determined lads found space for not just one, but a few pints apiece before the pub closed.

Why is it that we find ourselves eating to excess on some evenings, while other times we can summon the willpower to stop when we've had enough?

The Power of People

By now, it will come as no surprise just how many things in our environment influence what and how much we eat. Social and environmental cues both play a role in whether we eat too much or just enough, as well as how much we enjoy the experience either way. But what about the people at the table with us? What influence do our friends and family play in our eating behavior, and how do our socially influenced behaviors differ from the way we act when we're dining alone?

In order to understand the influence of our dining companions on our eating behavior, we can turn to the work of health psychologist John de Castro. In the 1980s, de Castro began a series of dietary diary studies, and by the 1990s he had collected the dining diaries of over five hundred people. Each participant in the study recorded their daily meals and consumption habits, but also wrote down details about whether they ate alone or in the company of others. This information provided social context for the eating patterns and it turned out to be highly illuminating.[67]

What relationship might our consumption have to the presence of others at the table? One might imagine that people might eat more when alone, since the single diner is free of the prying eyes of others and able to indulge desires without being judged. On the other hand, a room full of people for a holiday meal would certainly seem to encourage overconsumption.

De Castro discovered that study participants definitely ate more in groups than when they were by themselves. The effect of family gatherings during holiday meals was significant. Experiments by other scientists have since confirmed these results and reached similar conclusions, showing people eating 40 percent more ice cream and 10 percent more macaroni and beef in the company of others than when they are alone. De Castro named the phenomenon he discovered "social facilitation." Eating with others doesn't just lead us to eat a little more food, it makes us eat a *lot* more food. This kind of influence is more than enough to bust any diet.

So what is it about dining with others that increases our consumption habits? De Castro and other researchers examined a range of possibilities, from hunger to mood to distracting social interactions, but none of them accounted for the extra calories. Sometimes, the obvious answer turns out to be the right one. In this case, studies eventually revealed that the overriding factor explaining the difference in consumption between eating alone and in a group was simply the extra time we spend eating when others are present. When we sit at the table longer, we are going to eat more food.

The holiday studies revealed that not only do we eat more with others than when we are alone, but the number of people we dine with matters. The larger the group, the longer the meal tends to be, giving us even more time to pack away the calories. This finding was put to the test, and in studies where the mealtime was fixed, larger parties ate no more than smaller ones. In one study, 132 participants ate either alone, in pairs, or in groups of four. The scientists gave them either twelve or thirty-six minutes to eat cookies and pizza. It turns out when our mealtime is fixed, the influence of the party number disappears, and participants all eat similar amounts of food no matter how many they are dining with. This experiment provided strong and clear evidence that longer mealtime is the key to greater food consumption in the context of social eating.

Feast or Famine

Is there anything better than the anticipation of a sumptuous feast with family and friends? One of the joys of dining with others is the freedom to order anything on the menu—or even everything on the menu. Observations of diners in an Italian restaurant found that the larger the dining party, the more pastas and desserts each person ordered. Before we have even taken the first bite, we know that we are going to indulge our desires and have plenty of time to laze around to finish it all. Such observations led food scientist C. Peter Herman to propose his "feast hypothesis," suggesting that we don't just indulge more because of the social environment, but that we socialize precisely so that we can all eat more without the guilt overindulgence would produce if we did it alone.

Context Matters

While time appears to be a key factor encouraging us to eat more, our social situation does, at times, affect how and what we eat. Studies have shown that obese children ate *less* in groups than they did when eating alone. On the other hand, they ate *more* in the company of other overweight youth. Other studies found that women, in general, eat less in the company of men than in the company of other women.

These patterns suggest that in many situations we pick up our cues of what is appropriate behavior from those around us and eat accordingly. And these influences are not limited to how much we eat.

The Drive for Difference

The higher our socioeconomic status, the more we are torn between the need to fit in and the desire to stand out. We want to be unique, but not too different. We want to be part of the in-crowd, but not one of the masses. It is often a delicate balance between the two.

How much do others influence your decisions? Do you look around to see what others are doing or make decisions based on your own preferences and tastes? I think most of us would say that our choices reflect our own individual likes and dislikes much more than the influence of those around us.

Consider this situation: You go out to a nice bar with a group of friends. Everybody is laughing and joking and having fun when the waiter shows up and asks for your order. You had been eyeing the kale salad and the fish and chips, but in the end decided that you are really in the mood for kale. Case closed. At least it was, until one of your friends orders the same kale salad you had settled on. Then a second friend orders the kale salad. When the waiter gets to you, what do you do? Order the salad you had planned on ordering like everyone else, or switch to your backup dish, which had been quite tempting anyway, as you recall. What will it be? Are you a leader or are you a follower?

There is ample research from social psychology and consumer behavior to show that our decisions and judgments are influenced by the choices and decisions of those in the group that surrounds us. In Chapter 6 when discussing "the folly of the crowd," we talked about the research of Solomon Asch, which showed how powerful the drive to converge on a single answer can be. However, the restaurant situation is quite different; there is no particular requirement that diners converge on a single choice. While there is no objective right answer when it comes to food preferences, we often behave as if there is.

Behavioral economists Dan Ariely and Jonathan Levav wanted to know how people would behave in a restaurant group setting like the one described above. Would they opt to follow their personal preference, go along with the crowd, or switch to the next best option when their preferred choice was selected by someone else?[68]

Ariely and Levav conspired with the manager of the Carolina Brewery in Chapel Hill, just outside the campus of the University of North Carolina. Dressed as waiters, the scientists approached groups of patrons as they were seated and offered them a free sample of beer. Who could refuse?

Diners chose from a selection of four beers under two conditions. In the first, the waiters went around the table asking each person in turn for their selection. In the second setup, the waiters had the patrons make their selection privately, so that their decision would be independent of the choice of others.

How do you think people responded? Did people choose differently in the two situations?

Indeed, they did. The researchers found that when patrons ordered publicly, one by one, the group ordered a greater variety than when patrons ordered privately. It turns out people don't follow the crowd in such situations. Instead, they adjust their selection to make a unique choice.

While the diners might not all have gotten their first choice of beers, they did get free drinks. And the choice of what beer to get was theirs. They simply valued being unique more than getting their beer of choice. Everybody should have ended up happy, right?

Alas, standing out from the crowd in such situations may make you unique, but it doesn't necessarily make you happy. Diners in the groups that made a public selection reported enjoying the beers *significantly less* than those who chose privately. While it is not surprising that people who passed on their first choice might not be as pleased with their selection, it is striking that so many people would sacrifice their enjoyment for a little credibility with friends and coworkers.

The Wisdom of Crowds

Getting together with friends and family is a source of great joy, but it can also be a source of unwanted calories and hoppy beer. Once again, we find that the choices we make are influenced by invisible factors that, for the most part, we aren't even aware of. We overconsume in a crowd, and we are unnecessarily influenced in our choices by the decisions of others. By recognizing these tendencies, we can regain control of the situations and minimize the negative impact of our environment.

Next time you find yourself out to dinner with friends, be sure to order exactly what you want even if someone has already called dibs. And, if nobody else wants dessert, but you'd really like to have something, you can do that too. This should make you both happier and healthier.

Chapter 18

The Power of Social Influence

While working for the US Department of State, I enjoyed some amazing and memorable meals. There were lingering lunches in Italian cafés near the Spanish Steps in Rome, with course after course of pasta, meat, and salad, all washed down with wine and sparkling water, and there were rushed bowls of noodle soup slurped at a stall in a makeshift restaurant on the streets of Hanoi. During my thirteen years at the State Department, I traveled to dozens of countries in Europe, Africa, South America, and Asia, and in each place I experienced many unique dining customs that opened my mind to culinary possibilities previously unimagined.

This is what tourists do, right? You go to a new place and you take advantage of the opportunity to try new things. Similarly, when people move to a new a place, they often adopt the customs obtaining at their new home. When we take up residence in a new location and find ourselves surrounded by a new community, we tend to absorb the culture of the established society. This is hardly surprising. Much of the joy of living in a new country or community comes from immersing oneself in the local customs.

But have you ever stopped to wonder if your penchant for adopting these customs was by choice? Is it possible that we are being influenced, even manipulated, by the practices of others in a way that nudges us to conform to the group?

I have to admit that that certainly does not seem to reflect my experience. I've always felt that my adoption of local customs was a conscious decision. In fact, I would describe immersing myself in local customs as one of the great pleasures of travel. While my hosts may have encouraged me to try dishes that bordered on the alarming such as grasshoppers or deep-fried baby crabs from time to time, the fact is that despite the objections I may have voiced, I always thought it was in good fun. I never felt any real pressure to eat these things.

When I did push my comfort zone and try the sea slug, it felt like the right thing to do. I wasn't being manipulated; I was being drawn to the customs. At least, that's how it seemed.

Monkey See, Monkey Do

Culture feels like a quintessentially human creation and yet science is now realizing that many animal communities have cultures of their own. And, just like their human counterparts, animals, it seems, are prone to adopting local customs.

Evidence has been gathering for decades demonstrating that animals are capable of transmitting knowledge from one individual to another. Nevertheless, all the observational studies and the research with captive animals alike left room for doubt about the power of social learning in the wild.

In 2013, Dr. Erica van de Waal at the University of St. Andrews, Scotland, and her colleagues devised a clever study of vervet monkeys at the Mawana Game Reserve in KwaZulu-Natal, South Africa to test the concept of social learning in the field.[69] They wanted to know if culture could be learned and transmitted throughout a group of subject animals.

The scientists set out pink and blue corn in side-by-side plastic containers for four groups of wild monkeys in neighboring regions of the reserve. They soaked either the blue or the pink corn in bitter-tasting aloe leaves, with bitter pink corn provided to two groups and bitter blue corn for the others. It did not take long for the monkeys in each group to figure out which color tasted bad and to consistently avoid it.

After several months, researchers stopped treating the corn, so that now both the pink and blue corn were equally tasty and acceptable as food. The monkeys continued to avoid the formerly bitter corn.

Why Smart People Make Bad Food Choices

This was predictable conditioning, and it had been demonstrated in many studies previously, but van de Waal and her colleagues added a new twist to the study design. They wondered what would happen when new individuals—infants and immigrants—who had not experienced the bad-tasting corn were introduced to the groups.

What they discovered was that baby monkeys with no exposure to any bitter-tasting corn immediately adopted the color preferences of their mothers. Dr. van de Waal even observed the infants squatting on the rejected colored corn while eating the preferred, as if the rejected corn were not food at all.

The more interesting and surprising finding was that monkeys trained to eat only one color of corn and to reject the other quickly began eating the disliked-color corn when they moved into a group trained to favor that other color.[70]

The Power of Culture

If we think of culture as socially transmitted knowledge, skills, and information, we begin to see its influence in many kinds of animals. Culture is not quite so unique to people as we might have imagined.

So what, you might be thinking, if monkeys ignore or give up eating tasty food after observing another group's preference? What does this have to do with people, in general, and you and me, in particular?

Might it be possible for this research to tell us something about the motivations behind the customs we pick up while traveling abroad or visiting friends across the country and, more importantly, the customs that influence us every day at home?

The behavior of the infant and immigrant monkeys in the experiment suggests two different mechanisms at work in adoption of the local custom and preference for one color of corn over the other. The young monkeys learn from their mothers by observing which foods are good and which are bad. This is a clear example of social learning.

But the situation with the immigrant monkeys is different. They came to the new group with an existing understanding of which foods are good and bad based on their own experience. Social learning might have taught them that the corn they had been avoiding might not be so bad, but that doesn't explain the important fact that they also stopped eating the colored corn preferred by their previous group. Social learning taught them that the colored corn that had previously been rejected was now okay to eat. That left them with the knowledge that both colors of corn were now acceptable to eat. Social learning should have given them the option to eat both types.

The behavior exhibited by the immigrant monkeys does not appear to be social learning. Instead, it appears to be an example of social *influence*, which occurs when our attitudes, beliefs, or behaviors are modified by the presence or action of others. This can occur because of real or perceived pressure from the group or because we come to internalize the beliefs of the group.

Peer Pressure and Conformity

We tend to mimic the behavior of those around us. This social influence exerts pressure, sometimes overt and sometimes subtle, for us to conform our behavior to that of the group. That pressure can help to reinforce our best tendencies, or it can undermine them. Many bad habits, including smoking, drug use, and even obesity, spread through social influence.

Everyone who successfully navigated the hallways, gyms, and cafeterias of high school is familiar with the social influence known as peer pressure. At one time or another, we have probably all found ourselves on each side of the peer pressure equation, whether we find a friend encouraging us to stick around for one more drink or find ourselves prodding our kids to clean their plates.

Even without the overt urging or nagging that comes from peer pressure, we can still feel influenced to conform to the group. As we learned from the Asch study in Chapter 6, most of us would rather conform with the obviously flawed answer from a group of complete strangers than trust our own eyes. The power to conform is strong.

In this section of the book, we have talked about the power of the environment to influence our decisions. From the design of a menu to the layout of a grocery store, our foodscape is a powerful force guiding our food choices and reducing the role of conscious willpower in those decisions. For example, in one study, customers presented menus without "monetary cues" (i.e., "$" or "dollar") spent nearly 9 percent more than when the menus included the words or symbols.[71]

Taking the "Self" Out of Self-Control

It doesn't come as any shock to learn that habits like smoking and drinking are influenced by the crowd we hang out with, but obesity feels different. When we eat too much or fail to follow our diet plan, we tend to chock it up to a lack of willpower or self-control. However, as we saw in the last chapter, the foodscape extends to the people who surround us. Our social circle exerts an influence over us, even in the absence of the kind of overt social pressure that the Asch study amply demonstrated.

We generally think of social influence as undermining our willpower, but might it be possible for social influence to do the opposite and strengthen our will power?

In a series of studies, Dr. Michelle vanDellen of the University of Georgia and Dr. Rick Hoyle from Duke University discovered that both self-control and a lack thereof can be contagious, spreading by means of social influence through our networks. The researchers found that watching or even simply thinking about a person exercising self-control—in ways such as exercising, balancing their finances, or managing their food intake—can strengthen our resolve to stick with our fitness, financial, or food goals, or anything else that requires self-control on our part.

In one study, one group of volunteers stood by and observed while an individual chose to eat a healthy carrot from a plate in front of them instead of an appealing chocolate chip cookie from a nearby plate. A second group of the volunteers watched an individual choose and eat the cookie instead of the carrots. The individual who chose the carrots was meant to demonstrate "self-control," while the individual who ate the cookie was meant to be like the rest of us.

The volunteers had no interaction with the individual tasters other than watching them. The volunteers were later given tests to assess their own level of self-control. The researchers found that the people who had watched someone eat a carrot showed greater self-control themselves on the later test than those who had watched a person eat a cookie. The quality of self-control is evidently contagious.

Such studies do not give us an excuse to blame others for our actions, or absolve us of responsibility for our actions, but they do suggest that observing others can nudge us toward temptation or away from it. Social influence can make the difference between whether we choose to eat an extra cookie or stop by the gym after work. As vanDellen and Hoyle explain, "These studies should challenge the notion that self-control is only an individual struggle. People should be encouraged by the knowledge that their own self-regulation can influence those of others around them. By exerting self-control, people can increase the likelihood that others around them who take note of this will in turn be more able to exert self-control themselves. Likewise, when people consider whether they should exert self-control, they should be aware that failing to do so may not only cost them long-term benefits, but also that it might undermine the success of those around them."[72]

Why Smart People Make Bad Food Choices

Social Influence for Social Good

Too often today, social influence is making us less happy and less healthy. When we make decisions based on our social standing rather than our preferences, as we discussed in Chapter 17 in connection with the research of Ariely and Levav on beer selection, we end up less happy with what we get. And even worse, when we follow the crowd in ordering a dessert even though we're full or stick around for that drink we know we don't need, we not only undermine our happiness, but we also undermine our health. It is important to remember here that social influence nudges us, but it doesn't control us.

Meanwhile, the intriguing message from vanDellen and Hoyle's research is that if we can find a way to exert control over our own actions, it can not only benefit us, but it can and will help those around us do the same. We want to encourage good behavior, but often we unintentionally send an opposite message, particularly when it comes to eating. Too often, parents try to bribe their children by saying that they can only have dessert once they have eaten the vegetables on their plate. Kids aren't stupid. They conclude that if eating vegetables requires a reward, then it must be something they are going to hate.

Instead of bribing our children, we can exploit what we have learned about the beneficial power of social influence. We should be demonstrating through our actions that vegetables are good and tasty. As a parent, I know my children are watching me all the time. They are picking up countless cues about how and what to eat from my own behavior. They notice whether I fill my plate with vegetables or whether I just place a few token pieces on the side. They pick up on the fact that I always eat my vegetables first before turning to the meat on the plate. They know that if I do leave something on the plate, it won't be the vegetables.

An Intentional Foodscape

In Part I, we explored many of the ways our brains are leading us to make bad decisions, and in Part II we examined how the foodscape is conspiring to make us fat. Now it's time to consider what we can do about it. We can put all that we have learned to good use. In the next section, we will explore some exciting examples of the ways in which organizations and communities are getting their heads and hands around the need to reshape the foodscape. Foresighted pioneers and leaders are showing us that we don't have to passively accept the foodscape we discern around us. Equipped with our new awareness of how it all works, inside and outside our minds, we can design an *intentional* foodscape that will help to deliver better health every day. And most remarkably, we can have a realistic hope that we can make it do this without the need for us to follow prohibitively restrictive diets or give up the foods or the positive food experiences that give life so much quality and meaning. There is a brave new foodscape ahead.

By implementing changes in our own homes and communities, we can and will influence others to do the same. In Part III, we will learn how to harness social influence for social good in the foodscape. Let's get started.

Part III

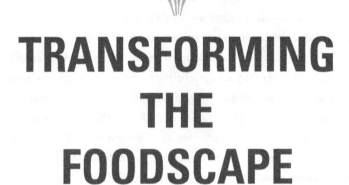

TRANSFORMING THE FOODSCAPE

A New Approach to Better Diets

In the first two parts of this book, we explored how our minds and our environment conspire to lead us to make bad decisions about the food we eat. Over time, these actions become engrained as habits, and habits are powerful things not easily influenced or altered by mere information or even our good intentions.

The traditional approach to dietary change is based on the notion that consumers respond to knowledge and information and adjust their behaviors accordingly. Doctors, nutritionists, and public health officials advocate for greater access to and transparency in information to reduce unhealthy food choices and prevent future illness. While it may seem self-evident that knowledge guides behavior, in Part II, we examined many instances where that simply doesn't happen. From package labeling to menu labeling, consumers consistently fail to take advantage of the information that is available to them. And when information is simplified to the point where consumers *can* take it into account, as with front-of-package claims like "low-fat," we see that consumers are just as likely to be misled by the information as to use it to make wiser food choices.

Despite the wide availability of vast amounts of information on how to eat healthy, most Americans have terrible eating habits that are contributing to the obesity epidemic undermining our health and crippling our healthcare system. This is a stubborn issue because of the psychology involved. Just as consumers are not influenced by nutrition information, they are not easily swayed by information about the risks of their current food choices and behaviors either. Most consumers already know that their eating habits are bad, and most would like to do better. We are constrained in our ability to change our eating behavior by habits, culture, and environmental influences. The problem is more complicated than a lack of information, and the solution will not be found in simply adding more information to the consumer's experience.[73] We must address these issues in bold new ways to achieve effective results.

It is beginning to look like accomplishing positive change in what we eat will have to do with more than the diets we choose to follow. Those willpower-based diets may not even figure in as a large part of the solution. We have long known that what we eat reflects a range of factors such as the cost of food, access to healthy options, knowledge of nutrition, our food preparation skills, time available for shopping, and time and energy to devote to food preparation. But what we are beginning to realize now is that our diet is also a reflection of our human environment, which includes social influences and pressure from friends, family and colleagues, advertising from food companies, and other cultural influences as well. All of these environmental influences could support positive dietary change, but too often, these factors oppose it, leaving us depending entirely on a dwindling reservoir of willpower.

We've tried changing our diets and public health officials have tried changing the information offered to consumers, and these measures have failed. It is becoming apparent that we have to find a different approach that is both more subtle and more powerful. We need to change our food culture.

Our foodscape may be the sum of all the food influences that surround us, but it is culture that solidifies their impact and locks them in place as habits. Culture is the foundation that underlies our food choices. Culture provides the rules that shape what we consider to be acceptable and preferable when it comes to food. It influences when and where and how much we eat, as well as what combination of foods we think go together and even what items are acceptable or unacceptable as food. While Americans may have a hard time thinking of insects as food, consumers in many countries find insects to be delicacies. My own experience eating tree grubs in Gabon and grasshoppers in Zimbabwe did not convince me of the virtues of these menu items, but I do realize that the disgust reaction I have to the idea of ingesting insects is based in my food culture rather than in an objectively repellent quality recognized by all societies. Custom and culture dictate many of our most basic ideas about what is good and bad. The ancient Greek poet Pindar rightly observed that "culture is king."

Our eating behaviors, conditioned by our food culture, are the accumulation of a whole lifetime of experiences, decisions, and actions. Changing them cannot be expected to happen overnight or even over the course of the weeks or months we normally stick to a new diet. In order to achieve lasting change in our behaviors and to establish new habits, our intentions must be reinforced by our foodscape.

Food policy experts like Marion Nestle have been saying this for decades, and yet the dietary guidelines continue to focus on getting consumers to reduce their fat intake or avoid certain foods or food categories. We have focused on fussy matters of food content and nutrition science rather than drawing upon the tremendous power that lies latent in an informed knowledge of relevant cognitive and social psychology. We have talked about habits and behaviors rather than behavioral science and choice architecture. But it's time for that to change.

In this third section of the book, we will look at how we can begin to reconfigure our foodscape to work for us instead of against us. We will examine some of the tools of behavioral economics related to "defaults" and "priming"—concepts that can be used to promote good behaviors without the active, or even conscious, participation of consumers in some cases.

We have each of us on average gained one or two or three pounds a year for the last thirty years to reach the point where two-thirds of Americans are overweight or obese. It has taken time to get here, and solving the problem will take time, too, but new approaches will lead us there. We can reshape our foodscape so that we begin to reverse the weight-gain trend.

Why Smart People Make Bad Food Choices

Can we really lose weight without effort by changing our environment? The idea seems too good to be true, and yet, as I will show you, there are already communities putting such ideas into practice. When our environment changes, our behaviors change as well because we have drawn on forces larger than our personal selves and the limits of our own willpower.

A review of these intriguing new experiments and some consideration of their successes will lead us to some thoughts on how we can begin to harness social influence to improve our health. We will consider what it would look like if society and culture were working with us in terms of food health rather than against us. The ancient Greek scientist-engineer Archimedes famously said, "give me a fulcrum and I will move the world." It may be that we are finding fulcrums that will dramatically alter our foodscape for the better.

Let's begin with a simple nudge.

Chapter 19

Food Nudges

Have you ever noticed how different grocery stores tend to have such similar layouts? Even competing grocery store chains often follow the same familiar plans, so no matter where in America you live, you've doubtless seen fresh produce along the perimeter and candy at the checkout aisles. A great deal of thought has gone into these layouts as stores attempt to maximize the profit value of our shopping cart by promoting mindless purchases. As we've learned, the positioning of sweets at the checkout takes advantage of the decision fatigue we all feel after slogging through the mental gymnastics of shopping.

Choice Architects

We saw in the first two parts of this book that people do not make decisions in a vacuum. They make decisions in the context of their environment, both physical and psychological, where many of the factors that influence their choices are hidden or invisible. Sometimes the environments we find ourselves in are deliberately shaped by other people, including the architects and managers who design our restaurants, grocery stories, school cafeterias, and even our homes. People who create environments that influence decisions are sometimes referred to as "choice architects." They are responsible for organizing the context in which we make our decisions.

Over the last fifty years, our environments have been recast in ways that promote unhealthy food choices and unhealthy lifestyles. All the willpower we can muster is not enough to overcome the power and momentum of our foodscape, railroading us into eating things we know we shouldn't. In this chapter, we begin to explore how the tide can be turned and the situation reversed. We will look at ways choice architecture can be used to encourage people to make better food choices and deliver healthier outcomes.

The goal is not to force certain outcomes on individuals, but rather to create environments that facilitate healthier choices. The tools of choice architects include "defaults," "feedback," and "incentives." These concepts were popularized in the 2008 bestseller *Nudge: Improving Decisions About Health, Wealth, and Happiness* by Cass Sunstein, a legal scholar, and Richard Thaler, a behavioral economist whose work won him a Nobel Prize in 2017. This interesting book explains why people don't always make rational choices, such as signing up for a 401(k) retirement plan when they start a new job, and how "nudges," such as making enrollment the default option, can help them make better choices. Nudge theory spans the fields of economics, psychology, and policy. It draws on a deep understanding of behavioral science to encourage people to make decisions that are in their broad self-interest, like retirement savings. Within the areas of health and food, it generally aims at encouraging positive behaviors rather than penalizing negative behaviors.[74]

Everything Matters

From the number of people at the dinner table to the size of our dinner plates, it turns out that many small and seemingly insignificant details in our environment can have major impacts on our behavior. As Thaler and Sunstein write, "A good rule of thumb is to assume that 'everything matters.' "[75] While economists like to think of us as rational actors making carefully considered decisions about what is in our best interests, behavioral scientists know that nothing could be further from the truth. We humans are subject to all manner of mistakes, including the biases we discussed in Part I of this book. We are bad at planning, self-control, and anticipating the future. Even when we are warned to be on our guard for such cognitive errors, we still make poor decisions.

Too often today, the designers of our foodscape, our food choice architects, are working against our good intentions to eat healthfully. Instead, they are conspiring with our intuitive minds to give us what we want rather than what we need, from convincing us to purchase the most profitable item on the menu or the extra appetizer. They play to our short-term interests, but these can very often diverge from our long-term goals.

Constructive Defaults

In Chapter 11, we contrasted two key parts of our brains—our intuitive and our rational minds. We learned that the rational mind is lazy and will often allow our intuitive to take the lead, which often means pursuing the path of least resistance. This tendency is often a source of consternation when we order the double quarter pounder over the salad. But what if the same forces that lead us astray could instead be harnessed for good? Our intuitive mind seeks out the easy answer not because it is bad or unhealthy, but because it is the one that comes to mind first. We can change what comes to mind first if we build a different environment.

Behavioral scientists point out that when people are given a choice, and one option is the default—the option that occurs if a person does nothing—then we can expect many, if not most, people to end up with that option, whether it is good for them or not. This occurs due to our bias toward the status quo—no decision is the easiest decision. If we can make the "better" choice the easy choice, we have one of those Archimedes fulcrums, and we can dramatically change our outcomes.

Defaults are ubiquitous and they are powerful. They can improve good outcomes, and they can also reduce the risk of bad outcomes. There are examples of constructive default thinking in garages everywhere: Most push lawn mowers in America today require the user to hold down a handle to start the motor and keep it running.

The same is true for chainsaws and many other power tools. So-called "deadman switches" stop the moving blades when the handles are released. Engineers have increased safety for the public by making these machines' safest condition the default. We don't have to rely on memory and willpower anymore to turn such things off immediately when our attention moves elsewhere. What if we could apply such constructive default thinking to our food environment?

Effective Feedback

One of the best ways to encourage people to improve behavior is to provide feedback. Unfortunately, when it comes to food, our bodies and minds don't do a very good job of giving us that feedback. In a perfect world, we would eat until we had had enough and then our stomach would send a message to our brain that it was time to shut our mouth down and stop eating. Instead, our bellies are slow to send that message, and often it does not arrive until long after we have eaten more than our fair share. By the time we typically get the message that we're full, we are more than full, we're stuffed.

The failure of immediate feedback is only half the problem. Not only do we often eat more than we should, but we don't eat the right things. This is also due to a lack of proper feedback. It is easy to think we can choose the greasy burger over the beans and rice bowl because we plan to balance out the indulgence of the moment with a healthier choice for the next meal. The problem with this is that the short-term negative effect is certain, while the long-term positive effect is only an intention—and too often it never actually materializes. Over the course of many days, weeks, and months, these decisions to engage in short-term culinary enjoyment at the cost of long-term health goals slowly take their toll. Sure, we see that negative results of these decisions eventually, but we can't tie them back to any specific decision. As a result, the feedback is diffuse and not particularly helpful when presented with another specific food temptation.

A well-designed food environment would present our choices differently. It would inform people when they are making good choices as well as when they are making bad choices in a timeframe that was relevant to the choice at hand. What researchers have found is that this is not nearly so hard as one might have imagined. A simple nudge can provide such feedback.

We can learn about food choice architecture from what has been discovered on America's roadways. Just as we ignore the food and menu labels that try to steer us away from unhealthy foods, we also too often ignore road signs that are meant to keep us safe. Transportation engineers track road accidents, so they are aware of sections of road and intersections that are particularly dangerous. They put up signs that tell us to slow down, or they flag a signal or a turn ahead that could put cars or pedestrians at risk. Despite such efforts, drivers continue to take corners too fast, sometimes with disastrous consequences.

Chicago's Lake Shore Drive is a scenic urban highway that twists along the coast of Lake Michigan. While the drive offers stunning views of the Chicago skyline, the scenic view coupled with tight curves makes for a dangerous combination. One particular stretch of highway was the source of many accidents for motorists who failed to heed the signs warning them to slow down. In September 2006, with the goal of reducing accidents, the Chicago Department of Transportation adopted a different strategy to slow the flow of traffic. Highway workers painted a series of lines perpendicular to the road and the traveling cars. The lines narrow as the drivers approach the tightest point of the curve, giving motorists the feeling that they are speeding up. The illusion of acceleration as the drivers approach the turn nudges them to reach for the brake and slow down.

The results were astounding. Over the six-month period following the introduction of the lines, crashes declined by *more than a third*. Emboldened by these results, the city implemented additional such changes that further reduced accidents and achieved a total decline across all interventions of *two-thirds*. This was a fantastic success record, with results in an arena that included life and death. It was an outstanding achievement, and it carries lessons that we can apply elsewhere for similarly positive results. What we learn from Lake Shore Drive is that rather than try to reach people's minds with more information, it is often better to reach them in the gut, where they will react first and think second. We speak to their unconscious mind, which is always apt to follow the easiest path, and we make that easy path the one that will lead to good results.

So how could this kind of feedback translate to the dinner table?

Portion control is a common recommendation for weight management. Doctors and nutritionists are constantly urging us to "eat less" of everything. While this may seem like a straightforward directive, given the realities of human psychology this scolding is unlikely to be the most effective approach to actually reducing a person's food intake. In Chapter 15, we discussed the impact of portion size on the rise of obesity in America. Getting people to eat smaller portions is hard given the value we perceive in large portion sizes. We know we tend to eat the food that is put in front of us, but reducing portion sizes without reducing plate sizes gives us the wrong feedback. Our brain looks at a partially empty plate and assumes we will be hungry at the end of the meal—producing the same feeling I had when served a double portion of food at the Cheesecake Factory on a plate triple the normal size. If you are going to serve smaller portions, you need to do so on plates that are appropriate frames for the portions.

Another option is to leave the plate size alone, but to manipulate the energy density or calorie content of the food. Nutritionists and doctors could encourage greater consumption of foods with a low energy density while keeping an eye open for high-energy-density foods. The great thing about this approach is that it relies on our normal way of deciding when we are full based on the volume of food consumed and how full it makes us feel. If we lower the energy density of our food, we will be able to eat the same amount of food, by volume, while reducing our calorie intake.

In one study, participants were asked to either eat more low-density foods like fruits and vegetables or to restrict portions. Those who had been counseled to eat more low-density foods lost 23 percent more weight. Interestingly, this group ate 25 percent more food by weight. They reported that they had less hunger and greater satisfaction with their diet than those in the other group.[76]

The Four Ps of Behavior Change

With books like Malcolm Gladwell's *Blink*, Daniel Kahneman's *Thinking Fast and Slow*, and Richard Thaler and Cass Sunstein's *Nudge*, the work of psychologists and economists in the behavioral sciences is reaching beyond academic circles to the general public. These books are about as far as one can get from the self-help and diet books for sale at the local coffee shop peddling some hot new diet trend. Steeped in the latest science about how people think and when they act, such books offer a new window into the tired subject of our poor eating habits.

In Part I, we considered the many ways our brains lead us astray, and in Part II, we looked at the influence of our environment. What we need now is not simply a list of the many ways things can go wrong or even a list of how things could go right, but rather a framework for acting on these insights. Fortunately, Zoë Chance, Margarita Gorlin, and Ravi Dhar, researchers at Yale University, have done the hard work and heavy lifting for us. They have distilled decades of behavioral science findings into a framework they call the **four Ps of behavior change** (process, persuasion, possibilities, and person), which provides strategies for making healthy choices easier and unhealthy choices a bit harder.[77]

Why Smart People Make Bad Food Choices

Process

According to the "four P" framework, **process interventions**, the first P, influence behavior by changing the position of options. This can occur in terms of the physical location, but also in the psychological realm in terms of an item's relative appeal or relative ease of selection. Process interventions for physical location include options for accessibility and order as well as the structure of the choice, as we discussed with defaults. Process interventions are quintessential examples of choice architecture.

When it comes to making food choices, the order with which we are presented with options is important. The first item in a buffet line or on a menu has a privileged status. It will receive more attention and be selected more often. When it comes to spoken options, as with the daily specials at a restaurant, the privileged positions are the first and the last items, which are often the only items we remember. This is simply the nature of human perception and memory.

Accessibility also has an outsized influence on our choices. This is why candy is often positioned at the checkout aisle, well within the view and reach of children. Small differences in accessibility or convenience—nudges—exert a gentle yet powerful influence on our choices. One study in a hospital cafeteria found that placing water at eye level in refrigerators and in baskets near food stations increased water consumption by 26 percent.

Persuasion

Persuasion interventions, the second P, change behavior by providing information or messages and then exploiting social norms that make healthy options more appealing and unhealthy options less appealing. Persuasive messaging is the sum of the information presented, the way it is framed and communicated, the moment when it is presented, and the person who delivers the message. Persuasion interventions are generally the least invasive and lowest-cost ways to nudge people toward better choices, since these nudges don't involve manipulating the environment. While the right message is critical, it must also be communicated in the right way and at the right time, when people will be most receptive to it. All these factors must be taken into account to construct an effective persuasion intervention nudge.

Possibilities

The third P is **possibilities**, which refers to the range of choices available or offered. Parents implement this intervention when they put vegetables on their children's plates. Unfortunately, the parents usually couple the offer of the healthy choice with poor persuasion messaging. While many parents find it tempting to attempt to bribe children into eating their vegetables with the promise of dessert if only they clean their plate, such an offer just confirms what a child fears, which is that the vegetable must taste pretty bad or parents wouldn't offer cake as a reward for eating it.

When changing possibilities, it's important to maintain freedom of choice. When New York City tried to ban large soda sizes, there was an enormous backlash, and not just from soda lovers. New Yorkers didn't like the idea of the government telling them what they could and couldn't drink. The negative reactions to the perceived paternalism drowned out the conversation about the potential health benefits of the policy. There's big difference between suggesting and banning.

When it comes to variety, our behavior is affected by perception as much as by reality—perhaps more. Studies have shown that people will eat more M&Ms from a bowl containing all colors than from a bowl containing only one color. It doesn't matter that all M&Ms taste exactly the same.

It is possible to reduce consumption of unhealthy food options without eliminating them altogether. One of the reasons we eat so much at holiday parties is because of the wide array of foods available. We feel the need to try each dish, which usually results in eating much more than we normally would. Eating a big serving of mashed potatoes, green beans, stuffing, and macaroni and cheese sounds pretty good. On the other hand, eating four big servings of mashed potatoes doesn't sound so appetizing.

Person

Process, persuasion, and possibilities allow choice architects to influence behavior in a specific context. However, the fourth P suggests that it is through the **person** that behavior can be influenced across contexts and over time. Changes to individual behavior are the most difficult to achieve and to sustain. It is not enough to change attitudes and intentions, since as we have seen, our behavior often deviates from our intentions anyway. Furthermore, our intentions are often not the problem. We have a pretty good idea of what we're doing wrong, we just don't know how to consistently do things better. We need better tools to help us.

We have discussed the limitations of willpower in several chapters. Decision fatigue and mental fatigue—as a result of hunger, stress, physical fatigue, or distraction—deplete our reserves of willpower. This is why motivation and willpower are not enough.

A more traditional approach to shaping behaviors is to set goals. Goals should be personal, motivational, and measurable in order for them to stick. By setting and tracking goals, we can begin to improve behaviors over time and slowly form habits. The majority of our actions are automatic, which means that *turning healthy behaviors into habits is the ideal way to sustain them*. We can avoid impulse purchases and eating through advance planning, such as preplanning or prepping healthy meals for the week. By setting goals and making plans and commitments to follow through with them, we can reduce the influence of our intuitive brain and bring more decisions under the control of our rational mind.

Implementation

What works in the lab does not always translate to the real world. Concepts that look good on paper may not be practical to deploy, especially at a large scale. Furthermore, implementing behavioral concepts in the home won't help us as soon as we venture out the front door. In order to build healthy habits for the American public, we need to have the entire national foodscape working to help us, not just the bubble that represents an individual home.

How do we convince governments, companies, grocery stores, restaurants, hospitals, schools, and other spaces where people buy or consume food to work toward these positive food choice goals and make changes that will promote public health?

One company has already taken the theories and tools of behavioral scientists to heart to improve the health of their workers, as we will see in the next chapter. If one company can accept the responsibility that comes with being a food choice architect, if they can adopt the strategies of the four P's and incorporate other lessons of nudge theorists, then perhaps we can succeed as a nation in creating a food environment that delivers personal health as the default. If we can spread the news of this exciting and encouraging development, other companies and organizations may have the confidence to follow suit.

Chapter 20

Googling Healthy Food

Obesity affects almost one in five children and one in three adults in the United States, putting them at risk for chronic diseases such as diabetes, heart disease, and cancer. The trend of increasing obesity has become a serious problem, and no effort to reverse it has worked.

Traditional public health campaigns, which specialize in telling people what they should do, routinely fail to alter the behavior that contributes to obesity. Since the early 1990s, agencies including the National Cancer Institute and the Centers for Disease Control and Prevention have been pushing their "five a day" initiatives to encourage Americans to get five daily servings of fruits and vegetables, but today, only 13 percent of Americans eat the recommended servings of fruit. Just 9 percent eat enough vegetables. The feckless corporate wellness industry—which offers health and fitness programs and incentives to corporate employees—has grown into an $8 billion behemoth without making much difference in the health of American workers or reducing corporate health care costs. And the dieting industry? The most successful results it generates are its $66 billion in annual revenue.

Health and wellness initiatives often fail because they place too much emphasis on providing information or gym memberships. As we saw in the last chapter, there is an extensive body of evidence from the fields of cognitive psychology and behavioral economics revealing that when it comes to food choices, information rarely succeeds in changing behavior or building better habits. Just telling people how to improve their eating habits may adjust their intentions, but in the food realm behavior often diverges from intentions. And many people, including many smart people, already know the things they are doing wrong. They have the information they need, but sadly, they feel powerless to do better with their diets.

The limited power of information to induce healthier decisions is especially evident when it comes to food choices. The need to make countless food decisions each day means we can't devote much processing power to individual choices. As a result, our eating behaviors tend to be habit- and instinct-driven rather than governed by good information. Just as our thoughts are driven by mental shortcuts, by biases and heuristics, our actions are guided by habits and shortcuts.

In Part I of the book, we learned some of the ways in which our brains undermine our efforts at self-control, such as through decision fatigue, or mislead us to unhealthy choices, as with the halo effect. Part II looked at the role of our environment, our "foodscape," in exacerbating the harm of our natural inclinations toward short-term benefits and simple solutions that drive bad food-related outcomes. With a clearer understanding of the operative influences on our food choices—context and impulsivity, for instance—we have a new opportunity to harness our habits and mental shortcuts and make them work for us rather than against us. We can devise measures and policies that will lead us to better food choices without us even having to expend extra energy and effort to get there.

The previous chapter introduced the concept of food nudges and presented examples of how we can harness these influences to make better food choices. We also saw, just as importantly, how individuals tasked with designing our food spaces can support our efforts. Now we will explore what it looks like to put these ideas into practice. This chapter examines a remarkable case study showing how one company, Google, effectively changed the food behavior of thousands of employees in their cafeterias and offices around the world. Impressive as this accomplishment is, improving the health of its employees is only the beginning of Google's ambition. The tech giant has its eyes on a much bigger prize, which is nothing less than helping to address the national and, with its global footprint, world obesity epidemic. The size and breadth of the company's operations ensure that their ideas have been tested at a large enough scale and with sufficient scientific rigor to provide useful data. Feedback and analysis have revised and improved their plans and decisions, and now Google is in a unique position to provide useful guidance to other companies that would like to implement such positive changes.

The Birth of Free Gourmet Food

Silicon Valley's tech giants are known for their free food. It isn't just any food, either. With their themed restaurants, gourmet menus, and stunning designs, the tech companies have elevated corporate dining halls above anything previously imagined. World renowned, Michelin-starred chefs serve up gastronomic delicacies at all hours of the day and night for the technology workers who have come to expect such pampering as the norm.

Google was at the forefront of this trend back in 1999 when the company hired its first chef, Charlie Ayers. With dishes like Sri Lankan chicken curry with roasted pumpkin served up fresh and hot to the rank and file employees at Google, it wasn't long before other Silicon Valley companies were compelled to compete with Google's legendary cornucopia of free food by offering up their own free smorgasbords.

A Man with a Mission

Google didn't set out to build a healthier way of eating. Cynics would say that the free food and snacks facilitated a culture of long hours and overnighters that benefited the bottom line at Google while taking a toll on employees. By raising the bar on food, the company made the daily grind a bit more palatable. Google cofounder Larry Page describes a different motivation for the food program. He had hopes of orchestrating "casual collisions" over meals that would lead to conversations that might not otherwise happen. Such cross-pollination just might lead to new ideas and new products for the company.

Over the next fifteen years, the number of employees at Google exploded, and the company was accordingly expanding its food service, not just in Mountain View, but in Europe and Asia as well. With a global operation feeding tens of thousands of employees every day in every time zone, Google came to need more than talented chefs. It needed someone who knew food operations and logistics on a massive scale.

In a 2020 article in *Wired* magazine, journalist Jane Black recounts how a phone call from a Google recruiter changed the life of Michiel Bakker. In 2012 Bakker was living in Brussels when the recruiter called about a new position the company was creating to oversee its corporate "canteens," as the cafeterias were called. The position might not have seemed an obvious fit for Bakker, who had fifteen years of experience opening and managing restaurants in ritzy hotels around the world, including St. Regis properties in San Francisco and the Pacific island of Bora Bora. He was nevertheless intrigued by the possibilities. "The role was to think through how to take food to the next level, to define what that next level would be."[78]

Bakker joined as Google's director of global workplace programs and has since been promoted to vice president. His first step was to reimagine the sterile corporate cafeterias as restaurants with inviting lighting, comfortable seating, and even a chef's table as part of an open kitchen so that employees could watch their food being prepared. These changes made Page's "casual collisions" less forced and more enjoyable. The new environments encouraged employees to linger and chat rather than inhaling their meals on the way back to their desks.

After the upgrading of the dining spaces, Bakker and his team spent the next year deciding what to do next. One problem they needed to contend with was the fact that employees loved the free food a little too much. New employees came to dread the "Google

Fifteen," named for the number of pounds they could expect to gain from a diet filled with fabulous meals, amazing desserts, and unlimited snacking and sodas.

It was about this same time that New Yorkers were engaged in a battle over soda cups. Then New York mayor Michael Bloomberg was pushing for a ban on large soda containers and receiving pushback from soda manufacturers, consumers, and retailers who sell the products. It's easy to see why people who make, drink, or sell soda might hate the ban, but the proposal also struck a nerve even among New Yorkers who didn't drink soda. For many people, the ban came across as a paternalistic effort to control people and tell them what they should and shouldn't drink. The measure failed, but it did highlight the very real problem of obesity in America discussed at the beginning of this chapter.

With this as a backdrop, Bakker and his team chose as their new focus the challenge of how to move Americans to a healthier diet while maintaining individual choice. He knew it wasn't going to be easy, explaining the problem this way: "The younger generation doesn't know food. They grew up in situations where family meals were not part of their daily lives, because both parents worked or for any number of other reasons. Even people who want to make great food choices don't know how. So, the question was, what we can do to help people make better choices—if they choose to do so?"

Intuitive Brain

Bakker's experience setting up restaurants and designing menus led him to work with chefs and food scientists in search of ways to get employees to crave healthier food the same way we desire a monster shake. Anyone who has struggled to choose the fruit cup over the chocolate chip cookie during the coffee break at a meeting knows that good-tasting healthy food is often no match for our cravings for indulgent foods. For far too many people, the intuitive brain will opt for the bacon cheeseburger over the portobello burger nearly every time.

This sad realization led Bakker to the conclusion that changing the food by offering tastier healthy options was not enough. He needed to tackle the foodscape. This meant rethinking the entire menu to ensure that nearly every option was healthy or, at least, reasonably so. But it also meant examining the spaces themselves and how employees used and maneuvered through them. In order to accomplish this, he was going to need help beyond the world of food operations and services.

Behavioral Science in Action

In 2012, Google reached out to the Yale School of Management's Center for Customer Insights to explore ways of helping Google employers make healthier food choices by applying the learnings of behavioral science. This partnership built on decades of research in cognitive psychology by researchers like Amos Tversky and Daniel Kahneman and behavioral economists like Richard Thaler and Cass Sunstein and put their teachings to the test in the crucible of the kitchens and canteens of Google offices around the world. The combination of academic research and real-world experience developed into the lessons of the "four P's of behavioral change" discussed in the previous chapter.

For the foodscape design that emerged, it was considered not enough to deliver treats that kept employees content and working hard; the food had to make them healthy as well. The campaign did not simply change the menu, but also took notice of how the food was presented. The Google Food team's tactics included limiting portion sizes and redesigning the food spaces to lead employees to healthy choices like water and fruit while discouraging the soda and candy that remained available. The goal, according to Michiel Bakker, was to make the healthy choice the easy choice and the preferred choice.

Why Smart People Make Bad Food Choices

Over the past five years, the company has taken exactly the sort of data-intensive approach to the food it serves that one would expect from Google. Methodical and iterative, Bakker and the Google Food team have created the largest and most ambitious real-world test of how to nudge people to make healthier food choices when dining and snacking.

Reimagining the Kitchen

In the previous chapter, we discussed how process interventions like accessibility can change the position or location of food options, impacting consumption patterns. Bakker wanted to find ways of encouraging employees to eat more healthy food and reduce consumption of unhealthy options, but he didn't want to eliminate completely the candy and snacks that Googlers had come to know and love, since they might revolt. He also did not want to go so far as hiding the candy in the broom closet. Instead, Bakker decided to conduct some experiments to see if modest changes to accessibility would deliver meaningful, or even noticeable, results. Fortunately, they did.

Larry Page had insisted on having snacks within a short walk of every Google employee. During the forty gruelingly long seconds it took for the coffee machine to brew a fresh cup, workers were left exposed to fruit, cookies, and lots and lots of candy in the break rooms, known as "micro-kitchens" in Googlespeak. The danger was compounded by the fact that the tech workers put in long hours. As we learned in the chapter on mental fatigue, people are significantly more likely to choose an unhealthy snack over a healthy one in such situations.

With the normal canteen setup, the snacks were positioned about 6.5 feet from the coffee machine. Bakker started his experiment by more than doubling the distance (17 feet) from the coffee. The few extra steps may not seem like much, but it had an outsized impact on snacking. That modest increase in distance reduced the likelihood of snacking by as much as 23 percent for men and 17 percent for women. For people like me, who drink several cups of coffee a day, this could be the difference between maintaining a healthy weight and adding a pound or two a year. It is exactly this slow trickle of weight gain year after year that has gotten most Americans to the place they are in terms of excess weight or obesity. In this straightforward experiment, Bakker was able to measure the impact of subtle design choices.

From the insights gained at the coffee station and from other experiments Bakker conducted, Google remade the 1,450 micro-kitchens at all of its global offices, applying the lessons learned. As a result, the bonanza of unhealthy snacks was pared down to M&M's and gummy bears, for the most part, which were positioned well away from the coffee machine. To further heighten the accessibility gap, they were concealed in opaque canisters or in a drawer. At the same time, healthy snacks were given primacy of place with a big bowl of fresh fruit sitting enticingly in the center of the counter nearest the coffee machine.

Bakker's team applied the same theory to beverages. The bottom half of the kitchen refrigerators' glass doors were frosted to hide the sweetened teas and sugary sodas. The top half were clear allowing Googlers to see healthy options like unsweetened spa waters, carrot sticks, and yogurt. Of course, the sweetened beverages are not truly hidden. Google employees know that those items are there behind the frosted glass, but not seeing them reduces the temptation to indulge. The powerful lesson: Sometimes a simple nudge is all it takes to change a behavior. It didn't really take much to turn a daily soda habit into a daily flavored water habit.

Building a Better Buffet

In Chapter 15, we discussed the American penchant for larger plates and supersized portions. Michiel Bakker was well aware of this trend and he took steps to address the portion size issue as well. While the Google cafés in New York, Athens and Singapore may look like the coffee bars, burrito shops, salad bars, and buffets you'll find anywhere else, they serve up one small change that makes a big difference. The standard dinner plate in the US has grown from nine to twelve inches over the last few decades, with recipe portions growing to fill the plate. By contrast, the plates at the Google buffet line are only eight to ten inches in diameter.

The positioning of items in the buffet line also determines what ends up on the diner's plate. As we discussed in the previous chapter, the first few items will be over-represented on plates. This is why vegetables always come first on the line. By the time employees get to the meat or the chocolate tarts, there's not much room on the plate to go hog wild with the less healthy choices.

Other changes play to the concept of unit bias. A burrito is a burrito, big or small, after all. However, a burrito at Google weighs in at about ten ounces, which seems pretty substantial until you're reminded that the Chipotle version clocks in at one pound nine ounces. The Google version is 60 percent smaller, and yet still more than enough to satisfy most people. Without the mega burrito from Chipotle as a comparison, we accept the ten ounces as an appropriate serving size.

According to David Katz, MD, MPH, founding director of Yale University's Prevention Research Center and president of the True Health Initiative, "What Google is attempting here is culture change. And that's the level we have to reach to transform behaviors and health for a lifetime." Through small, intentional choices, Google has rid a small corner of the world of some of the temptations that have driven the obesity epidemic. From twenty-ounce Caramel

Frappuccinos to Triple Whoppers, many supersized versions of food have been vanquished from the diets of Googlers, and most of the workers do not even notice they are gone.

The Bottom Line

The results of Bakker's experiments are impressive. In the kitchens of Google's New York offices alone, which feed more than 10,000 people daily, the company serves 2,300 breakfast salads every day, up from zero a couple years ago. Seafood consumption rose from thirteen to twenty-four pounds per person, a whopping 85 percent increase between 2017 and 2018. This occurred even though Google focuses on more sustainable but less popular species such as octopus, fluke, and shellfish. While soda consumption has remained flat at an average of twenty cans per person per year, water consumption has jumped sharply. In 2018, New York Googlers drank nearly five times more bottled water than bottled sugary drinks.

Paternalism

This is not to say that all Google employees appreciate the effort. The company has a famously open culture—albeit one that has faced recent challenges—that encourages employees to speak up, whether it's about Google's controversial artificial intelligence contract Project Maven or the decision to serve less meat. And Googlers do complain about the food. They snub the small glasses at the juice and smoothie bars. (Apparently, if you want more, it's too much trouble to carry two glasses.) Google eventually caved to a very vocal contingent's demand that the company start serving Red Bull in its New York office.

Bakker remembers a petition one Googler started to "cancel meat," which was quickly followed by another petition to "stop cancel meat" and then another to "stop serving kale"—which may or may not have been a joke. For his part, Bakker goes out of the way not to be seen as the food police. "As the employer, we are investing in the program, and we are dealing with your health care and your long-term health and well-being. But we very much believe in freedom of choice," he said. "So, we're not taking things away. There is no prescriptive: Thou shalt eat carrots." It's just that the environment has been subtly engineered to make carrots more appealing.

The Complexity of Food Choices

The idea of altering the environment to shift behavior is not new. Choice architecture, as we discussed in the previous chapter, is one of the foundations of behavioral science.

Food choices, though, are infinitely more complicated than one-off decisions like whether to enroll in a 401(k) plan. What you decide to eat is intimate, complex, cultural, and mostly unconscious. It depends on your personal tastes, your budget, what you pass on your way to work, whether your kids or spouse are picky eaters, and what your peers deem socially acceptable. Most essentially, it's driven by habits, which, as we know, are hard to break.

"In a data-driven environment like the one at Google, we still think it's the right thing," Bakker says. "Anecdotally, you can see it. You can feel it." And so, Google has plunged ahead, working with researchers to refine behavior science to address more complex scenarios.

According to Ravi Dhar, director of Yale's Center for Customer Insights, "Early choice architecture focused specifically on the process. You didn't change the set of alternatives, but you rearranged them." It turns out, you also have to make the vegetables more abundant and more compelling if you want to increase consumption.

The strategy seems to be working for Google. In one New York office, more than half the Googlers stopped at the salad station, conveniently located just inside the entrance. The buffet line

overflowed with vegetable dishes: an okra-coconut curry, followed
by roasted cauliflower with cashews, paneer cheese with tomato and
peppers, and a spicy tofu vindaloo. Sounds like heaven to me. The
only meat dish was lamb korma situated at the end of the buffet line.

The majority of Googlers filled their plates with the vegetable
dishes before they even arrived at the lamb. The employees acted as
if they were on autopilot as they scooped out the aromatic Indian
dishes, which is another way of saying they had formed a habit. A
handful of people deliberately kept their plates empty to have room
for the meat. A nudge is not about eliminating options or stigmatizing
meat eaters, it is about encouraging better behavior while leaving
ample room for choice and our inner sweet-toothed demons.

Taste Matters

In 2016, Google decided, for health and environmental reasons alike,
to steer more employees to the vegetables. The early push was not
as successful as Bakker had hoped. He knew they had the placement
of products right, and they could see progress that had come from
making the vegetables more abundant. But the lesson that took
Google the longest to learn is also the most obvious: If you want to
motivate people to eat their vegetables and like it, then they sure
better taste good. We eat the things we like and enjoy, not the things
we know are good for us.

Bakker eventually realized that making vegetables delicious is
not as easy. It takes a lot of peeling, chopping, and pureeing to coax
out the flavor. By 2018, Bakker was running out of patience, so he
turned for help to Mark Erickson, provost of the Culinary Institute
of America. Together, they created a plant-based cooking curriculum
that Erickson believes is "likely going to become the way we think
about and teach food and cooking in the future." The course was
rolled out in 2020. Instead of learning how to roast, fry, and sauté

meat, cooks are taught to roast, fry, and sauté cauliflower, broccoli, Brussels sprouts, and carrots.

Corporate Wellness

Google is not your ordinary company and its employees are not your average consumer. Google's parent company, Alphabet, is valued at nearly one trillion dollars, and its workforce is educated, motivated, and sophisticated. Still, the company's big experiment matters to a larger population than just the employees. The obesity epidemic in America is an existential threat to the well-being of every man, woman, and child in the country, and it is a problem that is rapidly spreading to the rest of the world. Public health campaigns to get Americans to eat more vegetables have failed miserably, and the food industry's marketing of diet foods, as we've noted, has benefited very little beyond the bottom line of the food companies themselves. Obesity and the associated health conditions that result from it are also overwhelming our healthcare system. Scientists, public health advocates, corporations, and schools are all desperately seeking ways to improve the American diet.

Bakker's approach at Google recognizes that there are no easy, one-size-fits-all solutions to the dietary challenges confronting employees or Americans. But to study the possibilities, Google has built the world's largest food laboratory, where they can experiment on 195,000 subjects. The experiment encompasses multiple meals a day, five days a week, in cities all around the world. Don't feel too bad for these lab rats. This lab is filled with unlimited spa water, sea salt chocolate chip cookies, kale salads, and other dishes that would be equally at home in a Michelin-starred restaurant.

Google does not brand its food program as "corporate wellness," but its objectives do fit the definition. The broader wellness industry has largely focused on interventions like gym memberships and weight management classes toward their goal of reducing employers' healthcare costs. Employee health would be a side benefit. The results have been underwhelming to say the least. A study published last year in the *Journal of the American Medicine Association* (JAMA) that tracked more than 32,000 employees at a large US warehouse retail company found that the company's wellness program failed to do almost everything it set out to do. According to Katherine Baicker, coauthor of the study and dean at the University of Chicago's Harris School of Public Policy, "If employers are launching a wellness program with hopes of a short-term or quick savings in health expenditures or absenteeism, this study should give them pause."[79]

So, are there any lessons to be applied from Google? Steven Aldana, CEO of WellSteps, a corporate wellness vendor, notes that Google is unique in its ability to offer employees such extensive benefits. However, he agrees that "to really improve health, you have to change behaviors long-term, and to change behaviors long-term, it takes a holistic, cultural approach." While the wellness programs did not translate into health care savings or reduced absenteeism as hoped, dietitians involved in the programs did describe dramatic changes in culture and perspective, such as healthier food choices in break rooms and more employees drinking water over soft drinks. Changes involved both employees and management of the company playing a role in facilitating the healthier options.

Perhaps expecting the programs to deliver changes quickly is a mistake. A holistic approach to food and health might work on the timescale and at the same pace as the problem it is trying to address. In other words, people became overweight and obese over years and decades. Wellness programs might want to rethink the timeframe necessary for the benefits to manifest themselves.

A Glimmer of Hope

Google's strategy of emphasizing the good and de-emphasizing the bad through behavioral interventions seems simple, but is it replicable?

The good news is that there are plenty of institutions that could follow Google's lead. That starts in Silicon Valley, where free food is the norm and where many Google Food alumni have taken up residence after absorbing a passion for healthy food from Michiel Bakker. But there also are ways these lessons could spread to the wider world. Google isn't doing it all alone. Giant food service companies like Compass Group, the largest food service company in the world, procure food, write recipes, and employ cooks who work at Google. Compass' food operations are extensive and varied, including corporations, museums, hospitals, stadiums, universities, even public schools. The company is already applying Google's strategies throughout its network. Maisie Ganzler, chief strategy and brand officer for a Compass subsidiary that operates food service at the Google headquarters, explains, "Google's research on the behavioral economics of naming plant-based menu items has directly influenced the guidance we give chefs throughout all our locations."

Meanwhile, the Culinary Institute of America plans to repurpose the plant-based curriculum it developed for Google to help individuals and other companies respond to consumer demand for delicious, healthy, and sustainable food choices.

Behavior-change strategies are spreading quickly to a variety of organizations beyond the walls of corporate America. School cafeterias may not be as famous as Google for offering the most appealing food selections, but if one considers the number of children involved, it is easy to see that the responsibility of these cafeterias for shaping the health of the American future is tremendous. Forward-thinking school food policy planners, who are seeing more and more obese students, are beginning to consider new approaches demanded by the unhealthy trends. The potential for coupling education about healthy food choices with the shaping and making of actual healthy food choices during the school day through low-cost behavioral-change nudges is an exciting frontier that offers much promise for the development of effective new strategies that can be copied nationwide from successful pilot programs.

Another important organization adopting behavior-change strategies to address diet issues is the US military. Lieutenant General Thomas P. Bostick (Retired) shared with me his experience and frustration as former Commanding General of the US Army Recruiting Command. America's ability to provide good recruits to the Army is being impacted by the obesity problem, and of course the situation is getting worse. Projections indicate that by 2030, a shocking 64 percent of potential recruits will not qualify for service because of their excess weight. In response to these findings, the military created a one-year demonstration program called the Healthy Base Initiative. The program retrained cooks, deployed menu labels, and experimented with moving the location of healthy and unhealthy foods. An assessment of the initiative found notable improvements in healthy eating. Notwithstanding the successful pilot, the fact remains that widespread implementation would be challenging due to complex procurement procedures and chains of command. We can nevertheless count it as progress that there is awareness of the fact that environmental factors can be deliberately altered to affect the food choices and the resulting health of our soldiers.

How to Scale

It won't be easy to remake the world in the image of a Google cafeteria, where big isn't necessarily better and kale is actually cool. But it's not impossible. The corporate wellness trend shows that companies will invest in ideas to improve health if a case can be made for a positive, or at least neutral, impact on the bottom line. Tech companies have also demonstrated their interest in making the health of their employees a goal through their food programs. These efforts are already being scaled through the work of companies like Compass that touch many organizations and industries every day.

However, aside from a handful of companies like Google where employees are consuming a majority of their meals at work, most people will inevitably leave the bubble of their hospital, school, or corporate cafeteria and find themselves in the real world, surrounded by supersized portions. The foodscape is bigger than any one company. In order for behavioral interventions to succeed over time, they must be integrated into our daily life and follow us wherever we go.

In the next chapter, we will explore efforts to take these ideas out of the corporate cafeteria and put them to work at the scale of communities.

Chapter 21

How to Live to Be One Hundred

Knowing that many of our decisions occur at a subconscious level, influenced by invisible factors that we don't recognize and that our environment is pushing and pulling us in ways that we can't easily discern, is one thing. Figuring out how to reprogram our thinking and reshape our environment to lead us to better health outcomes is quite another.

There is a saying, "If you want to go fast, go alone; but if you want to go far, go together." This saying applies to our travels, but also to our lives. If you want to live a longer and healthier life, you can't do it alone because so many of the things that contribute to a good life come from the world around us. A good life requires the help and support of an entire community.

What steps can we take to surround ourselves, or embed ourselves, in an environment that promotes health?

In the last chapter, we explored the applications of behavioral science to the foodscape at Google. The Google Food team, led by Michiel Bakker, applied the lessons developed in coordination with the Yale Customer Insight Center to promote healthy food choices. With nearly 200,000 employees eating multiple meals each day in this controlled environment, the Google experiment demonstrates that behaviors can change and people's lives can be improved with the right choice architecture. While not everyone will agree with all the actions taken by the food team, it's clear that the majority of employees are happy with the food options available and see the benefits of the program.

Other companies are taking notice of the potential of choice architecture to move consumers and customers toward healthier choices, including food service companies like Compass. With ach new kitchen and cafeteria that applies these lessons it increases the chances that the changes that occur will lead to the formation of new and better eating habits. The more people who shift their habits, the more likely social influence is to work in support of healthier behaviors rather than against them, which is the case today.

So, how do we go from a handful of tech companies with deep pockets providing healthy food to communities of healthy people?

It won't be easy. The trend toward unhealthy diets and more people overweight and obese is strong and has been moving in the wrong direction everywhere in the world for decades. Fortunately, there are some examples out there that provide a glimpse of what an environment could look like that is working on our behalf and nudging us to be our best selves. One intriguing approach is the Blue Zones Project, which grew out of two simple questions: where do people live the longest and why?

Blue Zones Project

The village of Villagrande in the province of Ogliastra on the Italian island of Sardinia sits more than 2,100 feet (700 meters) above sea level. On January 1, 2010, there were 3,441 inhabitants of the village living the same traditional lifestyles and engaged in the same agropastoral activities they had for decades.[80] Despite the fact that until the 1960s the region was among the poorest on the island, the people shared one common trait. They lived a very long time. Demographers Michel Poulain and Giovanni Pes and their coauthors published research on their findings in 2004, naming the regions with extreme longevity "Blue Zones."[81]

National Geographic fellow and world adventurer Dan Buettner took these findings and the work of researchers on other communities of long-lived people around the world and ran with it, publishing a bestselling *National Geographic* cover story, "The Secrets of Longevity," in 2005.[82] The people of Villagrande were unusual in leading long lives, but they were not entirely unique. A number of researchers had identified other communities of people that shared the longevity characteristic. Buettner explored a community of members of the Seventh-day Adventist church in Loma, California and the inhabitants of Okinawa, Japan. He wanted to know if the reason for their long lives could be identified. He went looking for the traits that contributed to their unusually long and, importantly, healthy lives.

Over the last decade, Buettner has elaborated on these findings in a series of bestselling books, starting with *The Blue Zones: Lessons for Living Longer From the People Who've Lived the Longest,* that examine the behaviors of people living in the Blue Zones and continuing with books that focus on traits like happiness and diets.[8384] As Buettner explains in his books, people living in these Blue Zones are outliving us not because they have figured out some secret to a long life that is hidden from the rest of us, but because they are actually doing the things we all know we should do. This means consistently eating a healthy diet and moving around about every twenty minutes or so during each day.

All we have to do is eat right and move more. It sounds simple, but Buettner says it took him years after that initial discovery to understand why the rest of us—who have heard this advice many times—are getting the simple diet and exercise formula so wrong.

Longevity Happens

In an interview with Hilary Brueck in *Insider,* Buettner explains, "People start thinking that the entrance way to a healthier lifestyle— for most Americans—is through their mouths. But the core tenant of Blue Zones, and it took me about ten years to realize what I'm about to tell you, none of them have better discipline, better diets, better individual responsibility, they don't have better genes than us." Instead, "they live a long time because longevity happens to them," Buettner says.[85]

What does "longevity happens" mean? It sounds a bit like new age, hippy mumbo jumbo (not that there is anything wrong with that).

Up until now, we have mostly been talking about the ways our brains and our environment conspire to deliver bad decisions despite our good intentions. Buettner suggests that the people living in these Blue Zones are not gifted with superior genes or willpower that allow them to reject the supersize option at McDonald's. They aren't leaving half the food on their plate when they feel full or opting for the kale salad over the rack of ribs. They aren't relying on choice architecture to keep them on the path to a healthy diet.

Blue Zone residents in Italy, Japan, Costa Rica, Greece, and California live in a world where healthy choices are the easy choice or the default choice. They move consistently through each day because they have things to do and places to be that require them to walk and move. Importantly, they also live lives with purpose and surround themselves with friends and families they help and who help them in return. They do need to be choice architects because they live in worlds that already possess a healthy architecture.

Changing our behaviors in isolation is hard. Our environment tests us at every turn, enticing us to return to our old habits. According to Buettner, "If you want to live longer and be healthier, don't try to change your behaviors, because that never lasts for the long run. Think about changing your environment." Of course, that's what the choice architects at Google are doing, but they don't have control over their employees' foodscapes when they walk out the front door of the office.

Putting Theory into Practice

Buettner wondered if it was possible to reverse-engineer a Blue Zone based on the lessons he gleaned investigating the original sites. In other words, could a community reshape itself into a place that made people healthier rather than sicker by making the right choice the easy choice? In 2009, he put his ideas to the test in his first Blue Zones Project in Albert Lea, Minnesota.

For the 18,000 residents of Albert Lea, that meant finding ways to get their bodies moving more consistently and eating more healthy food. Buettner encouraged city leadership to redesign parts of the city so that healthful actions were also the simplest choices. In response, the city added ten miles of sidewalks and bike lanes for its residents, and local businesses stepped up to make it easier to pick and eat healthy food.

The residents responded to the changes as Buettner had hoped. People started walking more, setting up groups that promoted community to reinforce behavior. Collectively the residents of Albert Lea shed four tons of weight (an average of 2.6 pounds per person). Similarly, a smoking cessation program led to a decline in smokers from 23 percent of adult residents in 2009 to 14.7 percent in 2016, resulting in $8.6 million in savings in annual health care costs for employers. The outcomes were not merely the result of broader societal trends as the county surged to thirty-fourth place in the Minnesota County Health Rankings (up from sixty-eight out of eighty-seven counties).

Buettner has now successfully trialed this environment-focused approach in a number of cities and towns across the United States. The results have been equally impressive.

From his initial success in Albert Lea, Buettner went on to consult with dozens of other Blue Zone Project cities around the country. It might seem expensive to build bike paths and sidewalks just to get people moving more, even if it does lead to some weight loss in a community. But for cities implementing these changes, the benefits are not theoretical or intangible, they can be measured in dollars and cents.

In 2013, Buettner championed an ecosystem approach in the city of Fort Worth, Texas, that reduced the smoking rate by 6 percent.

This single outcome saves Fort Worth an incredible $268 million annually. Related Blue Zone initiatives throughout the city likely save tens of millions of dollars more in other health care costs.[86]

America's Fattest City

Blue Zones and the work of Buettner with American cities may seem like an anomaly, despite the success in a number of locales, but similar programs implemented by other organizations have found similar success.

Sometimes the same idea will pop up in different places at the same time. Around the time that Buettner was launching his project in Albert Lea, Huntington, West Virginia had the distinction of being America's "fattest city" with an obesity rate over 45 percent. British chef Jamie Oliver showed up to fix the town as part of his television series *American Food Revolution*. Despite a combative tone that portrayed the school district food service director as the villain, Oliver's arrival succeeded in starting a much-needed conversation.

Recognizing that the city could take a more active leadership role in the health of the community, it installed more walking and running paths. The mayor helped set the pace and encouraged others to join him during his Walks with Mayor around town. While Oliver crafted recipes the school district could not afford and, by some estimates, students didn't like, the school district stepped up and revamped lunches and nutrition education in ways that worked for the community. A new farmers market, featuring local produce, became a community staple.

Promoting change by shaming local leaders is not an approach that should be replicated. However, Oliver did nudge the city of Huntington to find their own path. The city and community bought in to the need for change and, ten years later, the rate of obesity had dropped to 32.6 percent, a meaningful improvement.

Wellville

Founded by tech investor Esther Dyson and led by health-impact innovator Rick Brush, Wellville is a ten-year nonprofit project focused on equitable well-being. Dyson and Brush are supporting the efforts of five US communities in their efforts to improve health and well-being. The project has broader ambitions as well, as the two founders look to inspire other communities and promote change in how the nation invests in people, institutions, and systems to achieve equitable well-being for all Americans. It is a bold vision.

Wellville deploys advisors to support local teams in each community as they develop shared, long-term investment in people, institutions, and systems. The project also seeks to forge national partnerships to improve local capacity and advocate for policies, actions, and investments. The project conducts social and economic impact analysts to evaluate progress and a learning system that cuts across the communities so they can share lessons learned.

Contagious Behaviors

There are many other projects operating at various scales around the world, from a researcher-led community-wide program in Somerville, Massachusetts, to a long-term project in France involving school and community, kids and parents, food and physical activity, education and action. When an idea's time has come, it is often hard to hold it back.

The projects share a similar focus on the power of people coming together with their community to create change. What we don't find in the Blue Zones that arose naturally, those that Buettner and his team are trying to recreate, or in the projects by Jamie Oliver or Esther Dyson is an emphasis on any of the traditional American tools of healthy living, such as fad diets, personal trainers or detox treatments. There are no calls for greater self-discipline or the counting of calories or steps. The secret to longevity seems to be to live in a culture that leads to the right choices without anybody noticing.

Culture, in a broad sense, is cultivated behavior. It is the totality of our learned, accumulated experience which is socially transmitted, or in other words, behavior through social learning. The problem with corporate wellness programs and even Google's grand experiment is that people leave the health and wellness bubbles of the programs at the end of each day and they return to American culture. Just as the monkeys in the corn experiment quickly adopted the norms of their new group, Googlers and others are faced with the need to conform when they find themselves in the midst of a culture that has fewer guardrails for our unhealthy tendencies.

Buettner, Oliver, and Dyson each recognized the importance of community and culture to reinforce behaviors that could make us healthier. They understood that good behaviors can be just as contagious as bad behaviors when you reach the tipping point.

Elements of a Healthy Lifestyle

Dan Buettner distilled the ideas he uncovered from his travels and that he applies in the Blue Zones Projects into nine lessons which he describes in his bestselling book, *The Blue Zones: 9 Lessons for Living Longer From the People Who've Lived the Longest*.[87] Building on those lessons as well as the lessons from each part of this book, I propose a different paradigm for better living. The elements of a healthy lifestyle relate to how we think, eat, move, engage, and thrive, with a recognition that our environment is influencing each of these factors every moment of every day. I have summarized each of these elements below.

Think. Be mindful of the mental shortcuts and habits that lead to bad choices. Don't rely on willpower to overcome these tendencies. Instead restructure your foodscape to make the right decision the default decision. For example, always shop for groceries with a list.

Eat. We live in a world of supersized portions and ubiquitous food. Prioritize quality over quantity. Lead with vegetables. Set aside the portion to take home before you take the first bite. If you're a family of four, consider ordering three meals and share. If you're hungry at the end, order dessert without guilt.

Move. Always be on the move. Walk to the store, garden, do housework, do stuff. Fill your days with activity. The more we do, the more we feel like doing. People living in Blue Zones have active lives that keep them moving throughout the day. Of course, the flip side of moving is finding time to slow down and relax. Meditate, do yoga, pray, or take a nap, whatever relieves the stress for you.

Engage. Find time to connect with family and friends. People with strong, fulfilling relationships live years longer than those without. Get together for dinner or happy hour. According to Dan Buettner, being part of a faith-based organizations can add fourteen years to your life. Relationships and connections give our lives meaning, which makes us happy. Happiness and health go hand in hand.

Thrive. Find your purpose. Purpose gives us a reason to get up in the morning and something to look forward to when we go to bed at night. You don't have to be a surgeon to feel good about what you do. It's enough to part of something bigger than ourselves. The difference between the person who serves people in a restaurant and the person who serves constituents in Congress, is that the former sees the results of their work each day.

Environment. Our foodscape acts on each of the above element all the time. It consists of the food labels that distract us with claims of gut health to the lighting and music in the restaurant that prods our food choices and how fast we eat. It's not enough to be aware of these influences. We need to find ways of changing our environment so that it can nudge us toward healthier choices. Look for ways to reshape your foodscape at home and find places to eat and shop outside the home that are working with you and not against you when it comes to healthy eating habits.

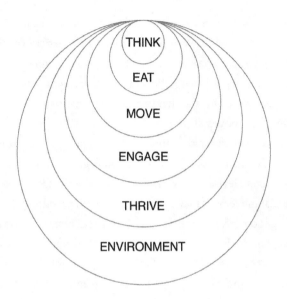

Keeping in mind the simple elements of a healthy lifestyle can have a profound impact on total quality of life.

Chapter 22

Scaling the Effort

In order for our food environment to begin to deliver health benefits we will need to revamp food culture in America. That's a big challenge and not one that can occur through public service announcements or targeted policy interventions alone. Ideally, the public will advocate for the changes, rather than oppose them as paternalistic or the results of the "nanny state." Change at the societal level occurs through the coordinated effort of people, organizations, and government. We have seen examples of change at the corporate and community levels, now we need to scale the change and turn it into a social movement that cuts across the entire foodscape.

The good news is that there are efforts underway that rise above the level of individual actions like mindful eating and corporate initiatives like the four P's for behavior change adopted by Google, and seek to promote change at the level of an entire industry. Let's start where most meals start, at the grocery store.

Healthier Lives

Grocery stores are a marvel of modern choice architecture. From the layout of the stores to the design of the signs, every item is exactly where it should be. From our discussions of nudge theory to the practical experience of the Google Food team, we know that these decisions by the stores' choice architects impact what we will purchase and, with that, what we will have for breakfast, lunch, and dinner. For the most part, these influences are invisible, but, given the placement of candy in the checkout lanes, we can guess our health is not an overriding consideration for their decisions.

Some retailers and food manufacturers are trying to change that. In 2018, a number of these companies came together in the United Kingdom to form a coalition—led by manufacturers and retailers

Why Smart People Make Bad Food Choices

and in partnership with public health authorities, local communities, academia, and other stakeholders—to explore new ways of addressing the obesity epidemic in the UK.

Together, the organizations established the Collaboration for Healthier Lives (CHL) to empower people to make positive changes to their health and well-being. The CHL Coalition's mission is to "inspire healthier behavior in stores, online and throughout communities around the world." The Coalition committed to helping people make healthier decisions every day in communities around the world.[88]

Recognizing the limitations of interventions based on information sharing and education, and understanding that eating behaviors are largely automatic, the Coalition turned to behavioral science for ideas. In other words, the Coalition encountered the same research discussed in the last two chapters, that what we buy and eat is an instinctive response to the environment around us. They targeted some of the same factors discussed in the four P's of behavioral change related to pricing and promotions, availability, choice architecture, and shelf and nutritional labeling as well as social feedback techniques. They wanted to apply the latest in behavioral science to improve consumer diets, not just in theory, but in a real-world grocery setting.

The results were impressive. Coalition companies trialed a total of thirty-four interventions using a number of the approaches to improve the healthiness of consumers' food baskets. The results showed a significant and positive impact on purchases. Following a year of interventions, stores observed consumers buying 13 percent more fruit and vegetables, 72 percent more beans, 19 percent fewer standard chips, and 22 percent fewer packets of confectionery.

The Coalition intends to continue and expand the interventions in more stores and more regions. This project not only shows that it is possible to nudge consumers to make healthier purchases under real-world conditions, but that businesses are willing to take steps to promote such outcomes. This runs counter to the common narrative that big food companies and grocery store chains want consumers to overeat to pad the bottom line and demonstrates that food retailers and food companies can be part of the solution.

The Power of Words

Words are important as we learned in the first part of the book. Consumers are often seduced by words like "natural" that carry a health halo that convince them to buy products that don't deliver on the health promise.

While words can be used by marketers to convince us to buy products that aren't really healthier, like organic cookies or candy, words can also be used to promote healthy foods, following the lesson of *persuasion* from the four Ps. In 2016, the World Resources Institute, recognizing that how we shop for food is predominantly based on habits, launched the Better Buying Lab to find ways for consumers to change their bad behaviors. To address this challenge, the Better Buying Lab develops strategies to motivate consumers to buy and consume more healthy foods. The lab brings together experts from consumer research, behavioral economics and marketing, and companies in the food industry to research, test, and scale new strategies and plans that help consumers select foods that are better for themselves and the planet. From these efforts, the Better Buying Lab produced a playbook to help food service companies support diners in choosing healthy, plant-rich meals. The playbook outlines twenty-three "behavior-change" strategies drawing on extensive behavioral science research into how people choose food, as well as insights from experts in the food service industry about what works and what doesn't.[89]

Panera Bread took a page from the playbook when they conducted a month-long naming test in January 2018. The chain's North Hills branch in California switched the "Low Fat Vegetarian

Black Bean Soup" to "Cuban Black Bean Soup" to highlight the origin of the dish and deemphasize its healthy nature. The simple change resulted in a 13 percent increase in sales of the black bean soup. The company's senior manager for Corporate Social Responsibility, Mindy Gomes Casseres, commented: "It was an exciting result for us. By showcasing the dish's origin, we were able to make the dish more appealing to guests. The new name conveys a well-seasoned and flavorful taste profile, and we think that's what led to a sales increase."

The playbook is designed to be used by anyone working in the food service sector wishing to make changes within their operations to encourage diners to choose healthy foods with an emphasis on those that are heavy on plants. The lab takes an approach similar to the Yale Center for Customer Insights, focusing on product, placement, presentation, promotion, and people.

The strategies outlined in the playbook should prove useful to a wide range of individuals in the food sector, including chefs, food servers, managers, salespeople, marketing and communications professionals, food operators, distributors, researchers, nutritionists, dietitians, and procurement teams. Together with the work of the CHL, these initiatives take behavioral insights from the grocery store to the restaurant, but also inform food companies developing and marketing healthier foods.

Nudge Units

Governments are increasingly turning to behavioral insights to promote public objectives by shaping the behavior of citizens and government personnel. A number of governments around the world have formed these so-called "nudge units," which are teams of behavioral science experts tasked with designing behavioral interventions that can encourage desirable behavior without restricting choice. Much of the interest in these approaches comes from the ability to test these interventions rapidly and inexpensively, before widely implementing the strategies that prove most effective. The United Kingdom led the way, establishing a nudge unit in 2010, and was soon followed by other countries, including Australia, Germany, The Netherlands, Singapore, and the United States.[90]

The White House established the Social and Behavioral Sciences Team (SBST) in 2015 to translate the findings and methods from the social and behavioral sciences into improvements in federal policies and programs for the benefit of the American people. During the two years the team was in operation, SBST conducted a number of interventions. One program aimed at increasing enrollment in retirement savings plans generated savings more than a hundred times larger than the impact per dollar spent by the government on tax incentives.

Growing awareness among governments of the potential of behavioral insights is encouraging, but there remains a large gap between the need for change in eating habits and the potential for behavioral science to accelerate that change. Governments must prioritize the creation of insights teams across departments and agencies. From the US Food and Drug Administration's Office of Nutrition and food labeling to the Department of Agriculture's Supplemental Nutrition Assistance Program and many others in between, the US government needs to ensure that behavioral science plays a central role in all decisions impacting consumer food, agriculture, and nutrition.

Engaging Consumers

The behavioral insights tools being developed for grocery stores and restaurants, corporate cafeterias and food companies touch a large portion of the foodscape that surrounds us. Each intervention builds on the work of others, reinforces it, and helps turn actions into habits. But these are examples of what others are doing to us. It is not only good, but essential that these businesses work with consumers rather than against them to make heathy food decisions, but we also need to do our own part. After all, a large number of food choices still remain in our hands and in our homes. We need to find ways of implementing interventions ourselves.

The lessons learned in Part I and Part II of this book help us do just that, but it is not enough. Sadly, not everyone will read this book. How do we bring all consumers into this virtuous cycle of supporting healthy food habits instead of resisting or even opposing the changes that companies are proposing? If consumers are not active participants in the promotion of changes to our foodscape and food culture, then it is quite possible they will oppose the interventions as unwelcome manipulation, just as New Yorkers opposed the ban on large soda cups as paternalistic and overreaching by the city government.

Social Context

As we saw in Part II, cultural influence and social context play an important our dietary choices, including what and how much we eat. Research has shown that traditions, beliefs, and values all influence food preferences. The type and quantities of food consumed are influenced by the people we eat with as well as the setting in which choices are made about what and how much to consume. Of course, cultural habits also change over time. For the last fifty years, they have changed for the worse. Perhaps now is the moment to begin to reverse that trend.

Food culture in the United States has changed dramatically over the last four decades and not in a positive direction. Many countries are tending toward a similar direction. The combination of excessive quantity and unhealthy types of food in restaurants and supermarkets, together with the lack of a suitable cultural and environmental context for reasonable consumption patterns, leaves consumers with no real guide for healthy eating. The most natural of human activities—feeding oneself and choosing what to eat—has become a herculean challenge requiring assistance from dietitians, food scientists, doctors, and social media influencers. Much of this advice is inconsistent and, at times, counterproductive, leaving consumers more confused than informed.

For too long, cultural and social influence have been negative factors impacting consumer food choices. In order to reinforce the efforts of grocery stores, restaurants, wellness programs, and other organizations that are crafting behavioral interventions outside the home to promote healthy choices, we need to find ways of bringing these interventions into our homes. Social support through families and friends can have a beneficial effect on an individual's food choices by encouraging and supporting healthy eating practices. Good habits, like bad habits, can be contagious. Behavioral interventions targeting cultural and social influence offer an entry point for the home.

Consumer groups and foundations have not yet leveraged social activism as a tool to promote behavioral change at the consumer level. The Better Buying Lab has its playbook for food service companies and the CHL has its report for the supermarket industry, however there is not yet a playbook for consumers or public interest groups. This book provides some practical advice for readers, but with two-thirds of Americans overweight or obese, we need to reach everyone. We need a social movement.

Starting a movement isn't easy. It is hard to mobilize society to address an issue, but not impossible. In recent years, we have seen people come together to tackle issues like pollution from plastic straws. While straws may not be as significant a problem as was originally thought, the point here is that society moved quickly once awareness was raised to mobilize change. Similarly, Americans rallied behind the ice bucket challenge which raised over $100 million for the fight against ALS (amyotrophic lateral sclerosis), a progressive neurodegenerative disease that affects nerve cells in the brain and the spinal cord.

Why Smart People Make Bad Food Choices

So, how do we get people to adopt behavioral change related to food? How do movements get started?

Don't Mess with Texas

We're familiar with the phrase, "Don't mess with Texas!" The slogan tells us something about the rugged nature of Texans, but do you know its origins? Who came up with the phrase and what was it originally used for?

Most people outside of Texas don't know how or why the phrase came into being, but it is fascinating story. It all started back in 1985. The great state of Texas, like many other states, spent a significant portion of its highway funds, nearly $20 million annually, to clean up litter along the state's roads and highways. The state tried fines and phone numbers for people to call to report offenders throwing beer cans and garbage from their car or truck windows, but nothing seemed to work. Texans seemed to love litter as if it was an expression of freedom. The Texas Department of Transportation was not so happy with this independent streak of Texans. Running out of ideas, the department eventually hired two ad executives, Mike Blair and Tim McClure, and tasked them with creating an ad campaign that would raise awareness, reduce litter and, most importantly, save the state money. It was a tall order, but the two were seasoned marketing men and ready to give it a try.

Blair and McClure eventually came up with an idea they thought fit the bill. They pitched the slogan "Don't Mess with Texas" to the Department of Transportation. It was not immediately embraced. Some thought it was too brash with one person suggesting they add "please" at the end. However, Don Clark, Director of the Travel and Information Division of the Texas Highway Department, thought the slogan was perfect. He felt it would speak to the eighteen-to-thirty-four-year-old male demographic most responsible for the problem. The "in your face" approach seemed destined to draw attention to the cause in a way that a more polite entreaty would not. Despite the transportation board's reluctance, Clark pushed ahead with the campaign, printing bumper stickers and highway signs and producing several television commercials. The rest is history.

Since its introduction thirty-five years ago, the slogan "Don't Mess with Texas" has taken on greater meaning for Texans, becoming a part of their identity (though the trademark of the Texas Department of Transportation). The campaign was also successful at reducing littering and remains one of the most successful ad campaigns of all time. The campaign highlights the power of the right message to mobilize people to action.

It Takes a Movement

Knowing what we should and shouldn't eat and knowing how to make the right choices are not the same thing. That's one of the lessons from behavioral science. I ended Parts I and II of this book with practical guides for putting the lessons from each chapter to use to improve food decisions. Many of the recommendations have been made before in books that promote a "mindful" approach to eating, which is another way of saying to keep in mind the mind's biases. Unfortunately, most of the articles and books on behavioral insights have been written as diet books rather than as books for everyone who cares about their relationship with food. Mindful eating isn't just about losing weight, it is about losing fear and stress and enjoying more of the food we eat. It is a lesson that is relevant to all of us.

Food is no stranger to movements. The organic food movement focuses primarily on the provenance of food and how it was produced. The Slow Food movement moves beyond food production to consumption and our relationship with food. Food culture determines if our habits are healthy or unhealthy.

Movements are not about sharing information. The CDC and USDA have been sharing information for decades about the importance eating five or more servings of fruits and vegetables a day. While most people are aware of this recommendation, only one in ten acts on it.

In order to start a movement, you need a few things. The first is a clearly articulated problem. In our case, the general problem is clear: too many people overweight or obese. But that is really a symptom of the problem created by a foodscape that is making us sick. It is the cause that needs to be addressed, not the symptom.

The second step is to identify the relevant stakeholders. This is also straight forward as we are all stakeholders in this problem since we all eat food. However, it is also helpful to break down the stakeholder groups into categories since they each have distinctive roles to play, including consumers, government, food companies, restaurants, grocery stores, agribusiness, academics, etc. It's a long list but not a complicated one.

Step three is awareness raising. In this case, the stakeholders are all aware of the problem and, for the most part, interested in doing something about it.

The fourth step is coordination and collaboration. This is where things begin to fall short. While many of the stakeholders are working on this problem within their respective silos, most of them are not connecting their efforts to other stakeholders. No group or organization has yet stepped forward to lead this effort or to bring these efforts to the consumer. Without leadership, we can't organize, and if we can't organize, we can't mobilize.

My Plate Challenge

What might such an intervention look like?

Human behavior is complex, but as we've seen with behavioral interventions in previous chapters, they can be targeted and effective. An obvious place to start with consumers is with the dinner plate. In Chapter 15, we discussed the evolution and expansion of portion sizes in cookbooks and restaurants over the last fifty years. Plate sizes have grown as well, from nine inches in 1960 to twelve inches today. That's more than a 75 percent increase in the area of the plate! Given that it takes about twenty minutes for the stomach to tell the brain it's full, which means many people finish their meal before they have gotten word from the stomach to stop eating. Since we can't rely on feedback from our stomachs, we determine the amount of food we can eat by estimating the volume of food on the plate. Some research suggests that if we use smaller plates and bowls, we will consume less. For that reason, many organizations, including the UK National Health Service, recommend using smaller plates to help people eat less food.

Restaurants might be open to providing smaller plates and portions if it didn't cut into their revenue, but the real danger is that diners would rebel or take their business elsewhere. While restaurants might want to adjust portions to promote health, from the perspective of many consumers, it might appear the move is to save money, which makes the eatery look cheap. Even if restaurants want to do the right thing, it isn't always that easy.

Telling people to use a smaller plate isn't much better than telling people to eat less. They might do it at home if they have a nine-inch plate, but what happens when they encounter the twelve or fifteen-inch monstrosities at restaurants? If we are constantly exposed to larger plates, our brains won't be satisfied with the amount of food served on smaller plates. The old way of promoting this message would have been through a public service announcement, but we know that information alone seldom works. Instead, we need social engagement to get the word out. Rather than make the smaller plate a personal challenge, we need interventions to promote social learning and social influence as a cultural challenge.

In the case of plates, this might mean encouraging people to take a nine-inch plate to restaurants. This might be embarrassing if you were the only one doing it, but it might be exciting to share the before and after photos on social media with the hashtag #MyPlateChallenge if friends were playing along. (I came up with this idea so feel free to be the first to post under the hashtag!) By coordinating such a campaign with organizations like the Academy of Nutrition and Dietetics, food influencers and others in the challenge could reach a broad audience.

Replating food allows people to see if the food served is a normal portion or extra-large. My experience with the outsized portions at the Cheesecake Factory discussed in an earlier chapter shows that the results can be pretty shocking. By replating the food, I not only avoided overeating, but got a second meal out of the visit. It was like getting two meals for the price of one.

Now, you might be thinking, is replating food really necessary? Perhaps you already divide your food in two on the plate, then take half home. It is a good practice, but we can do better. One limitation of leaving half the food on our plate is that our brains never get the signal that we're done eating. As we discussed previously, our brains need that signal to know it is time to start burning calories. By replating the food and then cleaning the plate, we signal the brain that we have, indeed, finished our meal. Second, if we simply eat half the food on our plate, we miss out on the opportunity to promote social learning and apply a little social influence of our own, which could nudge others to do the same thing.

Raising awareness of large portions could lead more people to set aside food to take home before taking the first bite. Restaurants might be more likely to participate in an effort driven by consumers. They could support the effort by offering diners the option of a half portion or perhaps a half portion on the plate and half to-go served at the same time.

The My Plate Challenge is just one example of how to mainstream behavior change. There are many more, but they must be scaled to be effective. The point is that a small intervention that draws attention to an important issue could generate interest in the broader issue of portion sizes in a more constructive manner rather than shaming people for eating too much or shaming restaurants for serving too much. The current foodscape often leads us to eat twice as much as we need. This outcome makes us less healthy and less wealthy. By tweaking the foodscape, we could find that we get two meals for the price of one or one full meal for half price and a healthier experience. Now, that's good value!

An Idea Whose Time Has Come

Over the last five decades, Americans have been inundated with nutrition information and overwhelmed by so-called health food products. The rise in obesity has coincided with the rise in diet books, cleanses, and food supplements, all purporting to offer solutions while the problem continues to grow. And yet, as challenging as the problem certainly is, I see reason for optimism.

The history of science is replete with examples of breakthrough discoveries that arose in different places at the same time. Charles Darwin and Alfred Russell Wallace independently advanced the theory of evolution, while Sir Isaac Newton and Gottfried Wilhelm Leibniz developed calculus. The phenomenon is even more common with many inventors sharing Nobel Prizes for their simultaneous discoveries.

A little over a decade ago, behavioral science made its way into the mainstream with books by Malcolm Gladwell, Richard Thaler and Cass Sunstein, and Daniel Kahneman. Fast forward to today, and nudge theory has moved from the lab room to the board room. At last, these ideas are making their way to government nudge units and organizations like the Better Buying Lab intent on applying behavioral interventions to public health. When it comes to bringing these efforts together to spark the cultural change necessary to deliver healthy outcomes, it seems like a question of when, not if.

The Lone Nut

I see the beginning of a movement, and I know this because I watched Derek Sivers TED talk, "How to start a movement," and it outlined the trajectory of a movement. Sivers' talk is perhaps the greatest three minutes on the TED platform. I encourage you to watch it, but if you don't have a computer close by, I will describe it.

Sivers shows a short video of a man in a park doing a crazy dance. The man dances alone for a while, but eventually someone joins in. Shortly after, the first two are joined by a trickle, then a flood of people joining the crazy dance. Within the span of the three-minute video, the park goes from relaxed sunbathing to hundreds of people frenetically dancing.

Sivers points out that the first few people who join are taking a chance, but by the time a group has formed, it becomes clear that something exciting is happening. As more people join in, it becomes less risky. Sivers' explains, "They won't stand out. They won't be ridiculed, and they won't be left out. If they hurry." Eventually, as more join, it becomes risky to stand on the sidelines since you might be ridiculed for not taking part. And that's how you form a movement.

Perhaps the most meaningful insight from the short video is when Sivers explains the importance of that first follower. Sivers puts it this way, "The difference between a lone nut and a leader is the first follower." We often underestimate the role played by the first follower, but later followers will be emulating that person, not the leader.

None of us have to be leaders in behavioral science. We just need to be willing to follow the science and become part of the movement. The trickle of resources currently flowing into these efforts will surge over the next few years, accelerating the pace of change. Governments, companies, and foundations that have been standing on the sidelines will begin to rush to be a part of this movement. After all, if they arrive too late, they risk being ridiculed.

It is up to each of us to look around and see how we can be part of the cultural change that will lead us as a nation to a new foodscape that promotes the healthy lifestyles we all want. By promoting nudges in our own lives and in the organizations and institutions that surround us, we can be a positive social influence on our friends, family, and community. The habits that changed to get us where we are today can change again. No willpower or grit required!

Chapter 23

The Billion Calorie Project

Our environment is part of the foodscape, but the foodscape also extends to our habits and culture. Good habits can improve health outcomes even in the face of a food environment that is tempting us to make bad choices. But it is easier if our environment and our habits are working together, rather than being at odds with each other.

In the last chapter, we looked at how social activism can scale behavioral interventions to the societal level. Ensuring that interventions are widely distributed is critical because that is how habits and culture change over time. One of the limitations of the behavioral interventions I've described so far is that it is often difficult to measure the impact in real-world settings. Even the Google Food team has found it difficult to measure the results of their nudges. If it were easy to identify one or two nudges that would have significant impacts on health, we would have identified them by now. The fact is that there are no silver bullets. We are subjected to hundreds if not thousands of invisible influences every day. Each nudge is guiding us to consume a few more or less calories. It is the aggregate of all of these nudges that determines if we consume too much or just enough.

Too often we try to lose five or ten pounds over the course of weeks or months, forgetting that that is not how we gained the weight, aside from the Google Fifteen or the Freshman Fifteen. Weight gain generally occurs slowly over the course of many years, one or two pounds a year for decades. If we can make enough small nudges to our foodscape, we can reverse the trend without even noticing the positive change and without any effort.

A Billion Calories a Day

The Billion Calorie Project is an idea I had that was borne from the notion that easy nudges that might have a tiny impact on each person can scale across society when implemented. More importantly, though, is the ability to quantify the reduction in calories consumed.

The project aims to identify simple behavioral changes that have the potential to reduce global calorie consumption by one billion calories a day. The changes could be implemented (or activated) through a social media campaign rather than policy changes. As a result, change could occur on a much faster timescale than what is normally required for nutrition interventions. The movement to ban soda straws demonstrates the potential of a social media campaign to ignite public engagement that can then be harnessed to effect change.

Soda Taxes Versus Nudges

Let's begin with a soda. Every day, consumers around the world visit hundreds of thousands of fast-food restaurants and consume tens of millions of cups of soda. If each person were to drink a few ounces less each day, billions of calories could be eliminated from our diets.

Taxes on sugar sweetened beverages (SSB) are a popular recommendation for reducing consumption. It's easy to understand the attraction. Taxes worked to dramatically reduce smoking, after all. However, while the United States' per capita soda consumption is among the highest in the world, consumption is at a thirty-year low. Proposals for SSB taxes have led to opposition in some jurisdictions. The taxes are generally opposed by restaurants and soda manufacturers, but also from groups pointing to the regressive nature of the tax due to its disproportionate impact on low-income households. Others oppose the taxes as paternalistic. Given the resistance, as well as a lack of direct evidence of taxes improving health, it is worth considering alternative approaches to reducing consumption that might receive greater support.

A behavioral approach to reducing SSB would look quite different from a soda tax. The goal of behavioral interventions is not to eliminate things that give us pleasure, but to ensure that we don't get too much of a good thing. It's hard to know when to stop drinking soda, and that's where nudges can help us. Rather than focus on forcing consumers to drink less soda by increasing the cost, it might be better to "nudge" consumers to drink less by changing soda consumption behavior in restaurants.

So, what might this look like in practice?

Size Matters

Instead of focusing on the price of soda, behavioral science offers other options. One of the most effective nudges relates to defaults. As we've seen in previous chapters, nudges can have a big impact on things as diverse as signing up for a retirement plan to willingness to be an organ donor. In the case of soda, the amount we drink comes down to the size of the cup. We also know that people tend to consume the food that is placed in front of them. That means if you drink from a big cup, you will drink more than if you had a small cup.

If diners order a small or large soda, then the default cup size is the one ordered. There are situations where the cup size is independent of the order and that is when people dine in a restaurant with free refills. If the default size is small, then diners will drink less. Having the small size as the default is different than banning large cups, as was tried in New York City. The option to request a larger cup remains.

Doing the Math

So what would it look like in practice if a restaurant chain switched the default cup size? Let's run the numbers on Subway, the largest restaurant chain in the world with more than 40,000 locations (McDonald's has about 37,000, if you're wondering). Subway restaurants commonly offer free refills to the 7.6 million diners served each day. For the sake of argument, let's assume they serve the same number of sodas.

The common default cup size at Subway is twenty-one-ounce (621 mL). A twenty-one-ounce Coca-Cola contains nearly sixteen teaspoons of sugar, compared to nine teaspoons in a twelve-ounce cup. By switching to a twelve-ounce cup as the default size, customers would reduce consumption by up to nine ounces (266 mL) per cup. Of course, customers will often refill their cup once before leaving.[91] If customers only get half a cup, that would be ten more ounces (296 mL) for the big cup and six (177 mL) for the small one. The difference between the big and the small is nine + three = twelve ounces (355 mL). A twelve-ounce Coca-Cola has 140 calories.

If Subway's 7.6 million customers were to receive the twelve-ounce cup as a default instead of a twenty-one-ounce cup, that would result in a reduction of more than a billion calories every single day. And that's only for one chain.

Counting Calories

A behavioral approach to the SSB problem offers some advantages over a tax. First, consumers may be more likely to support the smaller cup approach since they can easily request a larger cup if they prefer. Control remains in their hands. Second, restaurants may also be more likely to support this approach since they will actually save money by giving away less soda.

One of the limitations of soda taxes is that it is difficult to tell if the taxes are leading to health gains. You never know if consumers who drink less soda will switch to other sugary beverages or other snacks. Taxes in some cities have led to increased soda purchases in surrounding communities. Small default cup sizes are unlikely to result in compensating behaviors since consumers are unlikely to notice that they consumed less soda. This intervention would improve the bottom line for the company and the waistline for the consumer.

Win-Win Scenarios

Behavioral interventions offer unique opportunities to provide win-win outcomes for restaurants and consumers. The more you look for these interventions, the more obvious they become. Another easy intervention for Subway would be to separately wrap the two halves of their footlong sub. Consumers who finish the first half of the sandwich would be confronted with an unopened second half. Unit bias, discussed in Chapter 15, kicks in during such situations. Instead of viewing two half sandwiches, they would be more likely to view the meal as made up of two sandwiches. After finishing the first half, consumers would give serious thought to whether they should open the other half or simply take it home. Getting two meals for the price of one is good value.

Tackling portion control through defaults and other behavioral interventions holds great promise for our fight against obesity. Hopefully, others will be inspired by these straightforward ideas to propose and implement others. Together, we can begin to take a bite out of the obesity epidemic.

Conclusion:
Parting Thoughts

Why do smart people make bad food choices?

We've spent most of this book looking at the invisible forces that shape our thinking, from the biases at work within us to the foodscape that surrounds us. Most of the diet advice we get is focused on what and how much to eat. It's all about us as individuals. Food is deeply personal, after all. But we are not islands, and what we eat also affects those around us. We can readily see that our eating habits impact the choices and habits of our family and friends, but as we increasingly must recognize, the costs of overeating are also imposed on society as a whole. They can be measured in lives lost as well as in dollars and cents.

According to the *New England Journal of Medicine*, nearly 50 percent of Americans are expected to be obese by 2030 if current trends aren't reversed.[92] If we could maintain today's obesity rate of 42 percent—even though this is already a tragically high number—instead of reaching 50 percent, we could reduce future health care costs by hundreds of billions of dollars. Just as important, if not more important, is the cost to human potential. Our eating habits are not making us happy; they are killing us. 80 percent of major chronic diseases are preventable through changes to diet and lifestyle—eating a healthy diet, quitting smoking, and engaging in regular physical activity. This is not only an American problem, but rather a global epidemic.

The obesity epidemic is not about willpower and it is not about information. What has changed in the last fifty years is our foodscape. We are programmed to search for calories that used to be hard to find, but the mental shortcuts that served humans well in times of scarcity turn out not to be well-suited for the modern world of abundance. Everywhere we go, we are confronted with nudges to supersize our food or add bacon to our milkshake (an option at Five Guys, ugh!) and our brains simply shrug and think, "good value."

No individual person or organization is responsible for the mess we find ourselves in today. It was a collection of decisions and policies that may have seemed right at the time, but which have certainly not turned out well. The good news is that more people, companies, foundations, and governments than ever before are now laser-focused on the serious problem of public obesity. While some of these players continue to advocate for more information, many now recognize that it is the foodscape itself that needs to change.

There is reason for hope. In September 2020, the World Health Organization convened its first Technical Advisory Group on Behavioral Insights and Sciences for Health. According to the WHO, the creation of the technical advisory group is part of a new behavioral insights and sciences initiative, which is expected to give a more prominent role and louder voice to disciplines that have social and behavioral sciences in common in the context of health. The Director-General of WHO, Dr. Tedros Adhanom Ghebreyesus, noted: "Providing evidence-based advice is central to WHO's mission, but for that advice to produce results and save lives, we need to better understand the biases and triggers that affect whether or not people act on it."

I hope that you and the other readers of this book will find some practical lessons herein that will help you to improve the decisions you make. But this book is really a call to action for larger change because we can't address the public health crisis here and abroad alone. We need to change the world around us, and to do that we need to enlist all the stakeholders in the food system.

If we pay attention to our own biases and work together to build a new food culture based on behavioral insights, our environment can begin to nudge us toward healthy choices and, if we're lucky, we can rediscover some of the pleasure in our food that has been lost in recent decades. I hope that you will join me in creating that better food future.

Afterword

My goals for this book cannot be met without interaction and connection with readers who share my vision for a foodscape that works for us, not against us. In the effort to further a movement, every voice is valuable, encouraging others and pointing the way. A comment from you would strengthen the discussion, and I hereby invite you to post your own thoughts, however brief or lengthy, on my Facebook group page, @OurFoodscape.

I welcome reader feedback and would very much like to know what you think. If you have enjoyed this book or have ideas or suggestions to offer, please let me know at Jack@FuturityFood.com and help others find this material by posting a review on Amazon. com. You really can make a difference this way.

It is by engaging with one another and sharing our experiences, views, and concepts that we can move forward and create a healthier world.

Thanks for your time.

Endnotes

1 Svenson, O. (1981). "Are we all less risky and more skillful than our fellow drivers?" *Acta Psycholgica*, 47(2):143–148.

2 Zell, E., Strickhouser, J.E., Sedikides, C., and Alicke, M.D. (2020). "The better-than-average effect in comparative self-evaluation: A comprehensive review and meta-analysis." *Psychol Bull.*, 146(2):118–149. doi: 10.1037/bul0000218. Epub 2019 Dec 2. PMID: 31789535.

3 Fried, J. (2018, August 27). "Some Advice from Jeff Bezos." *Signal V. Noise.* m.signalvnoise.com/some-advice-from-jeff-bezos.

4 Leary, M.R., Diebels, K.J., Davisson, E.K., Jongman-Sereno, K.P., Isherwood, J.C., Raimi, K.T., Deffler, S.A., and Hoyle, R.H. (2017). "Cognitive and Interpersonal Features of Intellectual Humility." *Pers Soc Psychol Bull.*, 43(6):793–813. doi: 10.1177/0146167217697695. Epub 2017 Mar 17. PMID: 28903672.

5 This quotation is often attributed to philosopher and psychologist William James, but just because the internet says he said it, doesn't make it so.

6 Sutton, R. (2010, August, 27). "Strong Opinions, Weakly Held: Wisdom as the courage to act on your knowledge AND the humility to doubt what you know." *Psychology Today.* www.psychologytoday.com/us/blog/work-matters/201002/strong-opinions-weakly-held-wisdom-the-courage-act-your-knowledge-and-the.

7 Skubisz, C. (2017). "Naturally good: Front-of-package claims as message cues." *Appetite*, 108: 506–511. doi.org/10.1016/j.appet.2016.10.030.

8 doi.org/10.1111/spc3.12494.

9 www.marketwatch.com/story/amazon-could-redesign-whole-foods-stores-to-accommodate-online-grocery-delivery-orders-keybanc-2020-01-31.

10 Shiv, B., and Fedorikhin, A. (1999). "Heart and Mind in Conflict: the Interplay of Affect and Cognition in Consumer Decision Making." *Journal of Consumer Research*, 26(3): 278–292. JSTOR, www.jstor.org/stable/10.1086/209563. Accessed 19 Dec. 2020.

11 Vohs, K.D., and Heatherton, T.F. (2000). "Self-Regulatory Failure: A Resource-Depletion Approach." *Psychological Science* 11(3):249–254. doi:10.1111/1467-9280.00250.

12 en.wikipedia.org/wiki/Halo_effect.

13 www.readthesequences.com/The-Halo-Effect.

14 journals.sagepub.com/doi/10.1509/jmkr.43.4.605.

15 www.ncbi.nlm.nih.gov/pubmed/28853950.

16 onlinelibrary.wiley.com/doi/abs/10.1111/joca.12015.

17 Thorne, T. (2018, Aug. 22). "Produce and Pesticides in Perspective." *Sound Bites.* www.soundbitesrd.com/produce-pesticides-teresa-thorne.

18 link.springer.com/article/10.1186/s40550-015-0018-y.

19 journals.lww.com/nutritiontodayonline/Fulltext/2016/09000/Low_Income_Shoppers_and_Fruit_and_Vegetables__ What.6.aspx.

20 www.ncbi.nlm.nih.gov/pubmed/15479988.

21 Bobo, J., and Chakraborty, S. (2015). "Pink Slime, Raw Milk and the Tweetification of Risk." *European Journal of Risk Regulation*, 6(1): 141–144. www.jstor.org/stable/24323726?seq=1.

22 staging.foodinsight.org/questions-and-answers-about-ammonium-hydroxide-use-in-food-production.

23 Schlachter, B. (2012, April 14) "A Texas mom's fight against 'pink slime.' " Star-Telegram. www. star-telegram.com/living/family/moms/article3831060.html. Accessed January 11, 2015.

24 Gustavsson, J., et al. (2011) "Global food losses and food waste: Extent, causes and prevention." FAO. www.fao.org/3/a-i2697e.pd.

25 www.fao.org/save-food/resources/keyfindings/en.

26 Gates, B. (2012) "Annual Letter 2012." *Bill & Melinda Gates Foundation.* www.gatesfoundation. org/who-we-are/resources-and-media/annual-letters-list/annual-letter-2012.

27 webnesday.com/with-dan-barbers-dumpster-dive-experiment-table-scraps-get-celebrity-chef-treatment.

28 www.huffingtonpost.com/2015/03/27/blue-hill-wasted-pop-up_n_6949058.html.

29 www.coolhunting.com/food-drink/fine-dining-with-food-scraps-wasted-nyc-blue-hill-dan-barber.

30 Kahneman, D., and Tversky, A. (1984). "Choices, values, and frames." *American Psychologist,* 39: 341–50.

31 www.youtube.com/watch?v=jbkSRLYSojo.

32 Tversky, A., and Kahneman, D. (1974). "Judgment under Uncertainty: Heuristics and Biases." *Science,* 27: 1124–1131.

33 Mackendrick, N. (2014). "Foodscape." *Contexts,* 13(3): 16–18. ISSN 1536-5042, electronic ISSN 1537-6052.
    contexts.sagepub.com. DOI 10.1177/1536504214545754 journals.sagepub.com/doi/pdf/10.1177/1536504214545754.

34 Gladwell, M. (2004). *Blink: The Power of Thinking Without Thinking.* Back Bay Books.

35 Kahneman, D. (2004). *Thinking Fast and Slow.* Farrar, Straus and Giroux.

36 Kahneman, D. (2004). *Thinking Fast and Slow.* Farrar, Straus and Giroux.

37 Wood, W., Quinn, J.M., and Kashy, D.A. (2002). "Habits in everyday life: thought, emotion, and action." *J Pers Soc Psychol,* 83(6): 1281.

38 Price, C. (2017). "The Age of Scurvy" *Distillations,* 3(2): 12–23.

39 Mozaffarian, D., Rosenberg, I, and Uauy, R. (2018). "History of modern nutrition science: Implications for current research, dietary guidelines, and food policy." *BMJ,* 361:k2392.

40 US National Academy of Sciences Food and Nutrition Board, (1980). *Toward Healthful Diets.* National Academy of Sciences.

41 Pollan, M. (2007, Jan. 28). "Unhappy Meals." *New York Times.* www.nytimes.com/2007/01/28/magazine/28nutritionism.t.html.

42 Pollan, M. (2007, Jan. 28) "Unhappy Meals." *New York Times.* www.nytimes.com/2007/01/28/magazine/28nutritionism.t.html.

43 Pollan, M. (2008, Oct. 27) "In Defense of Food: The Omnivore's Solution." [Otis Lecture] Bates College. See www.bates.edu/news/2008/09/19/omnivores-dilemma.

44 www.mayoclinic.org/healthy-lifestyle/nutrition-and-healthy-eating/in-depth/paleo-diet/art-20111182.

45 Shostak, M., Konner, M., and Eaton, S. B. (1988). *The Paleolithic Prescription.* HarperCollins.

46 Spiegel, A. (2014, Apr. 14). "Mind over Milkshake: How Your Thoughts Fool Your Stomach." *National Public Radio.* www.npr.org/sections/health-shots/2014/04/14/299179468/mind-over-milkshake-how-your-thoughts-fool-your-stomach.

47 McClure, S., (2004). "Neural Correlates of Behavioral Preference of Culturally Familiar Drinks." *Neuron,* 44: 379–387.

48   Wardle, J., and Solomons, W. (1994). "Naughty but nice: A laboratory study of health information and food preferences in a community sample." *Health Psychology*, 13(2): 180–183. doi.org/10.1037/0278-6133.13.2.180.

49   Smith, K. A. (2013, May 30). "We have Texas to Thank for the Biggest Big Gulp." *Smithsonian Magazine*. www.smithsonianmag.com/arts-culture/we-have-texas-to-thank-for-the-biggest-big-gulp-84453489.

50   Mlodinow, L. (2018). *Elastic: Flexible Thinking in a Time of Change*. Pantheon.

51   Brownell, K., and Horgen, K.B., (2003). *Food Fight: The Inside Story of the Food Industry, America's Obesity Crisis and What We Can Do About It*. McGraw-Hill.

52   Wikipedia. (n.d.). *Super Size Me*. en.wikipedia.org/wiki/Super_Size_Me. Accessed November 16, 2020.

53   Rozin, P. *et al.* (2003). "The ecology of eating: smaller portion sizes in France than in the United States help explain the French paradox." *Psychol. Sci.*, 14(5):450–454.

54   Young, L.R., and Nestle, M. (2002). "The contribution of expanding portion sizes to the US obesity epidemic." *Am J Publ Health*, 92: 246–9.

55   Spence, C., Okajima, K., Cheok, A., Petit, O., Michel, C., (2016). "Eating with our eyes: From visual hunger to digital satiation." *Brain and Cognition*, 110: 53-63. doi.org/10.1016/j.bandc.2015.08.006

56   Pudel, V.E., and Oetting, M. (1977). "Eating in the laboratory: Behavioral aspects of the positive energy balance." *Int. J. Obesity*, 1:369–386.

57   Rolls, B.J., Morris, E.L., and Roe, L.S. (2002). "Portion size of food affects energy intake in normal-weight and overweight men and women." *Am J Clin Nutr.*, 76(6): 1207–13. doi: 10.1093/ajcn/76.6.1207. PMID: 12450884.

58   Rolls, B.J., Roe, L.S., and Meengs, J.S., (2010). "Portion size can be used strategically to increase vegetable consumption in adults." *The American Journal of Clinical Nutrition*, 91(4): 913–922. doi.org/10.3945/ajcn.2009.28801.

59   Benton, D. (2015): "Portion size: what we know and what we need to know." *Crit Rev Food Sci Nutr.*, 55(7):988–1004. doi: 10.1080/10408398.2012.679980. PMID: 24915353; PMCID: PMC4337741.

60   Food Insight. (2020, Mar. 9). *The Nutrition Facts Label: Its History, Purpose and Updates*. foodinsight.org/the-nutrition-facts-label-its-history-purpose-and-updates.

61   Chung-Tung, J.L., *et al.* (2014). *FDA Health and Diet Survey*. FDA Center for Food Safety and Applied Nutrition.

62   Niederdeppe, J., and Frosch, D.L., (2009). "News coverage and sales of products with trans fat: effects before and after changes in federal labeling policy." *Am J Prev Med.*, 36(5):395–401. doi: 10.1016/j.amepre.2009.01.023. Epub 2009 Mar 6. PMID: 19269126.

63   Bollinger, B., Leslie, P., and Sorensen, A. (2011). "Calorie Posting in Chain Restaurants." *American Economic Journal: Economic Policy*, 3 (1): 91–128. DOI: 10.1257/pol.3.1.91.

64   Gan, V. (2015). *New York's War on Salt*. City Lab.

65   Cantor, J. *et al.* (2015). "Five Years Later: Awareness Of New York City's Calorie Labels Declined, With No Changes In Calories Purchased." *Health Affairs*, 34: 1893–1900. 10.1377/hlthaff.2015.0623.

66   Petimar, J., Zhang, F., Cleveland, L. P., Simon, D., Gortmaker. S.L., Polacsek, M., *et al.*, (2019). "Estimating the effect of calorie menu labeling on calories purchased in a large restaurant franchise in the Southern United States: quasi-experimental study." *BMJ*. 367:l5837.

67   Herman, C.P. (2017). "The social facilitation of eating or the facilitation of social eating?" *J Eat Disord.*, 5: 16. doi:10.1186/s40337-017-0146-2 www.ncbi.nlm.nih.gov/pmc/articles/PMC5406877.

68   Ariely, D. (2008). *Predictably Irrational: The Hidden Forces That Shape Our Decisions.* HarperCollins.

69   Van de Waal, E., *et al.*, (2013). "Potent Social Learning and Conformity Shape a Wild Primate's Foraging Decisions." *Science*, 340(6131): 483–5. doi: 10.1126/science.1232769.

70   Belluck, P. (2013, Apr. 25). Monkeys are adept at picking up social cues, study shows. *The New York Times.* www.nytimes.com/2013/04/26/science/science-study-shows-monkeys-pick-up-social-cues.html.

71   Yang, S., Kimes, S., and Sessarego, M.M. (2009). "Menu price presentation influences on consumer purchase behavior in restaurants." *International Journal of Hospitality Management* 28(1):157–160.

72   VanDellen, M., and Hoyle, R. (2010). "Regulatory Accessibility and Social Influences on State Self-Control." *Personality and Social Psychology Bulletin*, 36: 251.

73   Nestle, M., Wing, R., Birch, L., DiSogra, L., Drewnowski, A., Middleton, S., Sigman-Grant, M., Sobal, J., Winston, M., and Economos, C. (1998). "Behavioral and social influences on food choice." *Nutr Rev.*, 56(5 Pt 2):S50–64; discussion S64–4. doi: 10.1111/j.1753-4887.1998. tb01732.x. PMID: 9624880.

74   Thaler, R., and Sunstein, C. (2008). *Nudge: Improving decisions about health, wealth and happiness.* Penguin Books.

75   Thaler, R., Sunstein, C., and Balz, J. (2013). Choice Architecture. In Shafir, E. (Ed.), The Behavioral Foundations of Public Policy. Princeton, New Jersey: Princeton University Press. pp. 428–39. www.researchgate.net/profile/C_Sunstein/publication/269517913_Choice_Architecture/links/548db1850cf225bf66a5f4e6.pdf.

76   Rolls, B. (2014). "What is the role of portion control in weight management?" *Int J Obes*, 38: S1–S8. doi.org/10.1038/ijo.2014.82.

77   Chance, Z., Gorlin, M., and Dhar, R. (2014). "Why Choosing Healthy Foods is Hard, and How to Help: Presenting the 4Ps Framework for Behavior Change." *Cust. Need. and Solut.*, 1: 253–262. doi.org/10.1007/s40547-014-0025-9.

78   Black, J. (2020). How Google Got Its Employees to Eat Their Vegetables. *Medium.* onezero. medium.com/how-google-got-its-employees-to-eat-their-vegetables-a2206820d90d.

79   Song, Z., and Baicker, K. (2019). "Effect of a Workplace Wellness Program on Employee Health and Economic Outcomes: A Randomized Clinical Trial." *JAMA*, 321(15): 1491–1501. doi:10.1001/jama.2019.3307.

80   Poulain, M., Pes, G., and Salaris, L. (2011). "A population where men live as long as women: Villagrande Strisaili, Sardinia." *Journal of Aging Research*, 153756. doi.org/10.4061/2011/153756.

81   Poulain, M., Pes, G., *et al.* (2004). "Identification of a geographic area characterized by extreme longevity in the Sardinia Island: the AKEA study." *Experimental Gerontology, Elsevier,* 39(9): 1423–1429. 10.1016/j.exger.2004.06.016. halshs-00175541v2. www.scribd.com/document/433365509/Blue-Zone-the-AKEA-Study.

82   Buettner, D. (2005, Nov.). "Longevity: The Secrets of Long Life." *National Geographic Magazine.* 2–27.

83   Buettner, D. (2012). *The Blue Zones: 9 Lessons for Living Longer from the People Who've Lived the Longest. National Geographic.*

84   Buettner, D. (2019). *The Blue Zones Kitchen: 100 Recipes to Live to 100. National Geographic.*

85   Brueck, H. (2019). "The man who unlocked the world's secret to living to age 100 says you can skip the gym." *Insider.* www.insider.com/blue-zones-dan-buettner-long-life-diet-exercise-2019-12.

86   Brueck, H. (2019). "The man who unlocked the world's secret to living to age 100 says you can skip the gym." *Insider.* www.insider.com/blue-zones-dan-buettner-long-life-diet-exercise-2019-12.

87   Buettner, D. (2012). *The Blue Zones: 9 Lessons for Living Longer From the People Who've Lived the Longest. National Geographic.*

88   The Consumer Goods Forum (2020). "Can supermarkets help turn the tide on obesity? A report from one year of the Collaboration for Healthier Lives in the UK." www.theconsumergoodsforum.com/global-learning-mechanism-resources/can-supermarkets-help-turn-the-tide-on-obesity.

89   Attwood, S., Voorheis, P., Mercer, C., and Vennard, D. (2020) "Playbook for guiding diners toward plant-rich dishes in food service." World Resources Institute.

90   Benartzi, S., Beshears, J., Milkman, K.L., *et al.* (2017) "Should Governments Invest More in Nudging?" *Psychol Sci.*, 28(8): 1041–1055. doi:10.1177/0956797617702501.

91   John, L.K., Donnelly, G.E., and Roberto, C.A. (2017) "Psychologically Informed Implementations of Sugary-Drink Portion Limits." *Psychol Sci.*, 28(5): 620–629. doi:10.1177/0956797617692041.

92   Zachary, J., *et al.* (2019) "Projected US State-Level Prevalence of Adult Obesity and Severe Obesity."
      N Engl J Med, 381: 2440–2450, DOI: 10.1056/NEJMsa1909301.

About the Author

Jack Bobo is the CEO of Futurity, a food foresight company that advises companies, foundations, and governments on emerging food trends and consumer attitudes and behaviors related to the future of food. Recognized by *Scientific American* in 2015 as one of the hundred most influential people in biotechnology, Jack is a global thought leader who has delivered more than five hundred speeches in fifty countries. He previously served as the Chief Communications Officer and Senior Vice President for Global Policy and Government Affairs at Intrexon Corporation. Prior to joining Intrexon, Jack worked at the US Department of State for thirteen years as a senior advisor for global food policy, food security, climate change, biotechnology, and agricultural trade. An attorney with a scientific background, Jack received a JD from Indiana University as well as an MS in Environmental Science, building on his BS in biology and BA in psychology and chemistry.

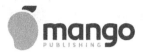

Mango Publishing, established in 2014, publishes an eclectic list of books by diverse authors—both new and established voices—on topics ranging from business, personal growth, women's empowerment, LGBTQ studies, health, and spirituality to history, popular culture, time management, decluttering, lifestyle, mental wellness, aging, and sustainable living. We were recently named 2019 *and* 2020's #1 fastest growing independent publisher by *Publishers Weekly*. Our success is driven by our main goal, which is to publish high quality books that will entertain readers as well as make a positive difference in their lives.

Our readers are our most important resource; we value your input, suggestions, and ideas. We'd love to hear from you—after all, we are publishing books for you!

Please stay in touch with us and follow us at:
    Facebook: Mango Publishing
    Twitter: @MangoPublishing
    Instagram: @MangoPublishing
    LinkedIn: Mango Publishing
    Pinterest: Mango Publishing
    Newsletter: mangopublishinggroup.com/newsletter

Join us on Mango's journey to reinvent publishing, one book at a time.

CPSIA information can be obtained
at www.ICGtesting.com
Printed in the USA
JSHW021121280321
12989JS00002BA/2